When Cells Rebel

Your Martial Arts and Defeating Cancer

This book was written for humans by humans.

Stickman Publications, Inc.
Seattle, WA 98126

ISBN-13: 979-8-9916023-0-3
First print edition

"Cancer... Nobody wants to hear that word, especially as you receive the diagnosis. Lots of things go through your mind when you hear those words. If you happen to be a martial artist, some of these thoughts run toward how you can continue training. What can you do, and so much more.

"The good news is that the authors have both been very long-term martial artists. Unfortunately, both have faced the dragon of the 'Big C.' This is good news. They share what helped them from the martial realm to navigate this new battlefield. From tips and tricks to ways of approaching your diagnosis, you are using the discipline you have trained. The philosophy of overcoming the odds in the biggest fight of your life.

"This is not a 'feel-good, it will be all okay' kind of book. It is a real, honest look at a crappy situation. The book is filled with wisdom and helpful advice from the front lines. Whether for yourself, or a person close to you, *When Cells Rebel,* will give you usable, caring, and understanding ways to maintain your balance and get through the BS that the diagnosis brings.

"Thanks,"

— **Terry Trahan** (www.patreon.com/WeaselCraft)

"My journey with cancer started in 2009. I returned from one of my several combat tours, this one after 13 months in Iraq. My initial reaction was, 'You have got to be kidding me.' I just had my annual flight physical and was given a clean bill of health.

"I was worried, I was concerned, but more than anything I was angry. How did I get cancer? I knew nothing about the thyroid, or what it did. So as with all challenges in my life, I took some time to reflect and ponder. After coming to terms with the situation and taking several long 5-mile-plus runs, three things came to me that put everything back into perspective:

"First, I survived several combat tours and for that I was grateful. Many did not, and some gave the ultimate sacrifice. Second, I had a fighting chance, and I needed to mentally, physically, and spiritually face this new challenge and work through it. Finally, cancer humbles you more than anything else. It brings you back to a place of reality and humanity. A long life is not guaranteed, but how you live your life is how you will be remembered."

— **Colonel Tim Fitzgerald**, USMC (Ret)

"Healthcare professionals are taught that a human is a complex entity with biological, psychological, sociological, spiritual, and cultural needs. Martial arts encourage the unity of mind, body, and spirit.

"In pursuing parallel journeys of health care and martial arts it has become evident that they share a mutual destination. That being good health and fulfillment in what form that takes for the individual. There is no doubt that in our pursuit of martial development, the mindset is essential. If you've taken a grade or competed, you'll know that mental preparation is essential for success. In healthcare, we see patients who positively approach their health challenges enjoy greater outcomes. Truly you can't separate the physical from the mental.

"This book will be inspiring and genuinely useful to the martial artist. Also, I suspect the non-martial artist facing their health battle will find this wisdom useful."

— **Peter Jones**, BN (Hons.) MSc RN (Adult)
Registered nurse
Emergency nurse practitioner
Advanced clinical practitioner
Oh, and *nanadan* in *Aiki-Jujitsu* plus lots of other accolades in which you'll (rightly) have no interest

When Cells Rebel

Your Martial Arts and Defeating Cancer

Kris Wilder &
Lawrence A. Kane

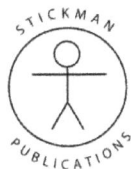

STICKMAN

PUBLICATIONS

Explore More Books from The Authors

Kris Wilder and Lawrence Kane are the bestselling, award-winning authors of *Musashi's Dokkodo, The Little Black Book of Violence, 10 Rules of Karate, Dude, The World's Gonna Punch You in the Face,* and *Martial Arts and Your Life,* among numerous other titles. Discover more below…

Kris Wilder

Lawrence A. Kane

"Cancer changes your life, often for the better. You learn what's important, you learn to prioritize, and you learn not to waste your time. You tell people you love them."

Joel Siegel

Table of Contents

Shadows gently fall

Murmurs of the
wind's last song

Peace in the nightfall

Preface

We want to keep this book crisp and useful, yet this story must be told. Richard "Rick" was a defensive tactics instructor. We both came to know him as one does in today's world, over the internet. We never met Rick face-to-face, but we talked to him over many years and believe that we knew his heart. You can find some of his insights in our book, *Martial Arts and Your Life*. Rick was brilliant, frank, and as cool as the other side of the pillow.

Cancer chased him. He was diagnosed with acute myeloid leukemia (AML), a rare bone marrow abnormality that damages a person's blood cells. As you might surmise, he didn't win that race. But he didn't run from cancer; he turned and drew his metaphorical knife (he liked knives).

Rick didn't prevail, yet this is not a story of defeat. Rick's is a story of dignity, clarity, and drive.

He approached his diagnosis with a stoic attitude. In our exchanges, he never moaned about his situation, and never complained. We never heard him ask, "Why?" Rick was never angry, not with us at least. He appeared to skip the stages of grief, or quickly integrate them, moving through denial, bargaining, depression, and anger, and then on to acceptance.

He accepted his situation, yet he also had a goal, to see his grandchild graduate from high school. Simply put, he adopted both a goal and a process-driven attitude. Rick had a purpose.

Cancer is confusing, frustrating, and unfair.

We as martial artists know that this is the way life works. There are few promises.

As Dave Pelzer wrote, "You can be a victim of cancer or a survivor of cancer. It's a mindset." Rick had the right mindset. He was a warrior, not a fighter. Warriors know when and how to go to war; fighters only know how to fight. Warriors may not always prevail, but they never give in, never give up.

We want to tip our cap to Rick. Rick was a friend. He helped us when we asked. He gave us input and inspiration as he stood tall in the storm of cancer.

There is a powerful lesson for us all as we face the gut-punch of a cancer diagnosis.

We are here to tell you that like Rick, you are a warrior. Victory is straight ahead. Meet every challenge with dignity and determination as he did. This is not nightfall, but the dawn of your most difficult battle.

Never fear. You are a martial artist. That means no matter what happens you're ready.

"One day in retrospect, the years of struggle will strike you as the most beautiful."

Sigmund Freud

Introduction

Mother Nature asked, "Who wants cancer?" I wasn't listening so I raised my hand.

Neither of us was paying attention that day when Mother Nature asked the question. We both survived. You have the same secret weapon we do, martial arts. The physical and mental strength that comes with your studies has built you for your fight. You already know discipline, grit, and determination, as we do.

A few numbers for perspective: The American Cancer Society (ACS) reported 1,958,310 new diagnoses in the United States in 2023. If you're male, you have a 1 in 2 chance of receiving a cancer diagnosis during your lifetime. For females, it's 1 in 3.

The most likely types of cancer we can expect to face vary by gender. According to ACS, the most common diagnoses[1] in 2023 included:

Male		Female	
Prostate	29%	Breast	31%
Lung & bronchus	12%	Lung & bronchus	13%
Colon & rectum	8%	Colon & rectum	8%
Urinary bladder	6%	Uterine corpus	7%
Melanoma (skin)	6%	Melanoma (skin)	4%
Kidney & renal pelvis	5%	Lymphoma (blood)	4%
Lymphoma (blood)	4%	Thyroid	3%
Oral cavity & pharynx	4%	Pancreas	3%
Leukemia (blood)	4%	Kidney & renal pelvis	3%
Pancreas	3%	Leukemia (blood)	3%
Other & unspecified	19%	Other & unspecified	21%
Total	100%	Total	100%

The good news is that roughly 6.5% of the population, some 21.5 million people, have studied martial arts in America, with about 6.9 million of them actively practicing at any given point in time. Some

---

1 Cancer can develop in any organ or tissue of the human body except for teeth, hair, and fingernails. It can also metastasize and spread beyond the primary site where it first develops. These statistics are associated with just those primary sites.

estimates suggest that there are well over 100 million committed practitioners worldwide. If you're one of them, and since you're reading this book chances are good that you are, you've been preparing to survive your diagnosis ever since you walked into the training hall.

You see, martial arts are competency-based. You've already learned how to set high expectations for yourself. You have persevered through adversity. You have felt the pride of setting and achieving challenging goals.

According to a 2019 Stanford University study, "The Will to Live," published by Ernest H. Rosenbaum, M.D., and Isadora R. Rosenbaum, M.A., the physical and psychological elements of the body are linked. As a martial artist, you didn't need a study to tell you that.

Importantly, their findings demonstrate that many cancer patients transcend their physical illnesses through a process of psychological revitalization. In other words, those with the strongest will to live have a better chance of doing so. As martial artists, we rarely lack willpower.

In that Stanford study the authors reported, "Many physicians have seen how two patients of similar ages and with the same diagnosis, degree of illness, and treatment program experience vastly different results." We could not find definitive evidence of exactly how one's attitude affects their outcome, there are too many variables, but it's clear that managing anxiety, pain, fatigue, nausea, and depression commonly associated with cancer diagnosis and treatment improves both a patient's quality of life and chances of survival.

In this book, we'll share the lessons we have learned from our cancer diagnosis, treatment, and recovery. In one case it was metastasized stage 4 adenocarcinoma, a type of cancer that starts in the glands that line your organs, and the other was myelodysplasia syndrome, a rare cancer that occurs when your bone marrow doesn't produce enough healthy blood cells. This work isn't about us, however, it's about you. We're sharing this with the trust that you will benefit from our experiences.

We're martial artists, not doctors, so we're not qualified to diagnose or treat anything. Nevertheless, we have a uniquely blended experience, as you do. We believe you'll benefit from the things we've discovered. At minimum, you won't have to figure them out the hard way. Getting through this requires a team. Know that we're on your side.

Kiritsu is a Japanese word that translates as, "Stand up." We're here to help you do that, just like we did.

One last note. In this book, we get to the point, have some inspiration, and don't wallow in the diagnosis. That was the disease's last free punch, now we return fire.

Tight

*Breath held in
constrained spaces*

Freedom lies beyond

Toilet Paper Tube View Doctors

The truth is that many doctors see you through a toilet paper tube, a narrow view. It is as if they took that tube and held it to their eye, close the other, and that's all they observe. Not every doctor sees you this way; we don't want to paint every medical professional with a broad brush, yet it is a common phenomenon in medicine generally and even more so in oncology. If you have such a doctor, in some ways it's an advantage. But, it's not gospel; you need to treat the information as their best assessment.

In most instances, you'll be working with a team, not a single medical professional. There are oncologists, surgeons, radiologists, hematologists, dieticians, and RNs to name a few. All the folks involved in your treatment will have different viewpoints based on their specialty and experience.

That toilet paper tube doctor is helpful, they are going to give you hard data and statistics. This is not a bad thing, but it is a narrow lens. To see the full picture of what you need to do to regain your health you'll need to reconcile the perspectives of your entire medical team, which sometimes means wading through conflicting information.

We're going to leave you with what Kris' statistics professor said at university. At the beginning of the class, he announced, "Statistics are a lot like a prostitute, you can get them to say and do anything that you want." Take the statistics, take the data, and use it. Don't let it crush you or create despair.

For example, according to the world's leading authority on myelodysplastic syndromes at Fred Hutchinson Cancer Research Center, Lawrence has been dead for seven years. That prognosis was incorrect. The facts from your toilet paper tube doctor are what you need and desire, but they must be used in conjunction with perspectives from other medical professionals for a comprehensive appraisal.

Doctors have informed opinions, but they're not omniscient. They don't know everything. It's called "practicing" medicine for a reason.

Between tall mountains

Narrow trail winds
endlessly

Horizons expand

They All Care

Cancer can be overwhelming not only to the patient but also to everyone around them. It's not something that most folks have been taught how to process let alone work through. Everybody cares differently, regardless of how challenging it may or may not be for them to express it.

Some people are compelled to bring food; others want to visit you. Some are afraid to make contact because they fear they might say or do the wrong thing. Or they're just uncomfortable with the diagnosis. Others reach out by phone or text. It's all good. Everybody has their unique way of expressing concern for you. You need to accept their version of caring.

Here's the professional move. When somebody says, "I wish that there was something I could do," or some version of that phrase, accept it and let them know that whatever they are doing is helpful, even if it's nothing more than reaching out. Know that they are encouraging you with their phone calls, visits, gifts, or whatever. They are doing the best they can do by expressing their concern over your situation. Acknowledge that and let them know that you appreciate them.

Everybody in your circle of friends, coworkers, and family who knows about your condition will be concerned about you, yet everybody cares in different ways and expresses their feelings differently. Acknowledging that they care is releasing for them. And, in many ways, also for you. In doing so you remove anxiety and that opens the door to even more positive experiences.

Victory's sweet breath

Heart and soul in
every stride

Champion's spirit soars

You're Not a Victim

A few days after my annual physical I got a call from the doctor. "Hey, it looks like we need to redo one of the blood tests. I've called it into LabCorp, would you mind going in tomorrow and having it done?"

"Sure, no problem."

A few days later, another call. "Would you mind doing one more test?"

"Um, okay."

A couple of days later, another call. "Would you mind doing one more test?"

"You're making me nervous. Is there something I should know?"

"Nothing to be concerned about. I'm just being thorough."

A week after that. "I'm not sure what to do with these results, so I'm going to refer you to a specialist, Dr. Ginsberg. Your referral should be approved by Monday and you can schedule an appointment then. His number is 206-..."

"I'll, um... Okay... I'll do that."

Monday morning, they answered the phone, "Seattle Cancer Care Alliance, how may I direct your call?"

"Fuck!"

Your diagnosis probably came as a shock, ours sure did, but it's important to understand that you're not a cancer victim. You're you. Sure, you have a disease, you have to deal with cancer, but you cannot let your disease become your identity. That's anathema to martial arts. We learn early on that while we're still breathing there's a chance to continue the fight. We don't give up, we don't give in. Win or lose we give it our all. With cancer it's no different.

Echoes in the wind

Words dance on
unseen currents

Bridges built in sound

A Safe Word for When You're Not You

You are probably going to be on many different medications. These prescriptions have side effects that can put you into a mental state that you are not accustomed to. Depending on the treatment(s) you're undergoing, you may experience everything from nausea to cognitive difficulties. While two patients undergoing the same procedures often have divergent side effects, some of the most common impacts of treatments include things like pain, fatigue, anemia, nausea and vomiting, and mouth problems such as difficulty swallowing, changes in taste, or hot/cold sensitivity, along with problems with your skin, hair, and nails.

In other words, due to physical or emotional side effects, you may well not be thinking straight, and you may not even know it. This is where the "safe word" concept comes into play. Your primary caregiver, your spouse, your adult child(ren), and even your nurse, will all need a safe word that they can use to point out when you're not yourself, one that you can acknowledge.

This safe word is designed to keep you on track and to allow others who have clarity of thought to act on your behalf. You will know that word as a pre-agreed-upon signal and at that point you will recognize the safe word and relax into the safety of those who have your best interests at heart.

In this fashion, you'll know when you're not being yourself, and have a chance to course-correct gracefully. It's challenging enough for those around you to care for someone who's being treated for cancer, and even more so when the treatment adversely affects your personality or outlook. This safe word concept helps you maintain an even keel in an otherwise tumultuous situation.

Pale moon through
thin clouds

Sickness casts its
quiet shade

Healing dawns anew

Alcohol Swabs Are Emergency Nausea Sniffers

Are you feeling nauseous? Since chemotherapy, radiation, immunotherapy, bone marrow transplants, and most other cancer treatments and drugs cause nausea, chances are good that you are. Is your medication for nausea not taking effect fast enough? That's common too. A simple hack for many patients is to sniff an alcohol swab. It does not solve every problem instantly, but it can take the edge off. It is that simple.

There are numerous "life hacks" for dealing with the side effects of your treatment such as sniffing alcohol swabs that patients discover. This varies from individual to individual, of course, but oftentimes there are commonalities that come with specific diagnoses and treatments. Consequently, it is valuable to connect with others in your situation. Knowing what works for them expedites the discovery of what works for you.

Cancer care centers, hospitals, and community organizations can connect you with support groups, workshops, websites, and social events that further your education and understanding of the disease you face while simultaneously helping you build a network of folks in the same situation who you can talk to about it. Look to organizations like Cancer Lifeline, Cancer Pathways, Cancer Hope Network, or the like to discover "cheat codes" associated with your treatment.

Additionally consider complementary medicine, such as naturopathic oncology, which is proven to enhance your quality of life during and after treatment and often improves your chances of survival too. Research indicates that combining conventional medicine with complementary therapies such as naturopathic medicine, acupuncture, acupressure, message therapy, meditation, or biofeedback improves outcomes for cancer patients.

In fevered twilight

Dreams blend with
waking sorrow

Recovery's light

You're Going to Throw Up on Everything

Get containers to put next to your bed, in your living room, in your office, or any room where you expect to spend time. Often you are going to feel the regurgitation coming on, and have time to react. However, there will be times when you will not, and it will be violent and unannounced.

Don't create extra work for yourself and others if you can avoid it. Cleaning sheets, clothes, vehicles, walls, and carpets is an additional problem that can be prevented with a little preplanning. If you can, do it. It'll create one less hassle.

A series of inexpensive plastic buckets or Ziploc® bags make all the difference. Ziploc bags? Yes, put one or two in your back pocket when you are out and about. They will serve you well if you become ill with little warning and there's no bucket or bathroom nearby.

This doesn't work for everyone, but many cancer patients find that inhaling the aroma of essential oils such as peppermint, ginger, or lavender, either from a container or by rubbing them onto your skin, can help with nausea. According to the National Institutes of Health, peppermint works the best for most patients. The aroma may not keep you from throwing up, but it often will give you a little more time between feeling the need and puking. Every little bit helps.

Stars guide weary steps

Night whispers
secrets of old

Horizons await

Everything is Incremental

As you know, the journey through the martial arts ranking system is a process. You have a goal, a challenging one like becoming a black belt or equivalent thereof that takes several years to achieve, but when you embrace the process, you won't get discouraged along the way. The process requires that you meet a variety of milestones that demonstrate your progress both to yourself and to your instructor(s), and these interim accomplishments are motivational.

The incremental mastery process in martial arts is designed to let you look back and see progress, and look forward and know exactly what's needed to get to the next milestone. Treating your illness is much the same as the rank passages you're familiar with in your training.

Your doctors have a process. Here is the issue, however: The doctors understand their process, the timing, the volume, etc., but you do not. It is all new to you and at times confusing.

Unlike the martial arts curricula which is explained to students when they walk in the door, doctors rarely describe what to expect in plain, everyday language that patients are sure to understand. And, you're likely reeling from the shock of your diagnosis, which clouds your understanding of what has been shared, especially early on. Consequently, you're likely to wonder why they are not doing more of what you believe they need to be doing or do it faster or more frequently.

We are not suggesting you passively engage in that process based on a lack of complete understanding of the process and plan. You must be active in your healing. You must embrace the process with the understanding that much of the experience is going to be an incremental progression.

It may feel like baby steps, but baby steps are fine. Your job is to understand what's going on, make sure you're pointed in the correct direction. Continue to make progress on your healing journey, moving forward one step at a time.

Morning light so warm

Grateful for each
dawn's embrace

Life's new start each day

Be Grateful

Not too long ago, your diagnosis was a death sentence. We live in a time today, however, where a cancer diagnosis is not a death sentence. That's a very good thing.

Emerging research, including discoveries from the Human Genome Project (HGP), various "cancer moonshot" initiatives, and ongoing research have led to breakthroughs such as immunotherapy, precision medicine, advanced radiation therapies, immune checkpoint inhibitors, nanomedicine, and gene editing. For example, it's possible to "reprogram" a patient's DNA[2] to eliminate their deadly bone marrow disorder with chimeric antigen receptor, or CAR T-cell therapy, a new immunotherapy.

New treatments are being invented and tested faster than ever nowadays. While the statistics vary by type of cancer, according to Cancer Research UK the overall patient survival rate has doubled over the last five decades. What was once uncurable is now treatable.

Statistics are great, but they apply to the typical, average, median-modal person. That's not you. In other words, it's not just medical advances that matter, it's how early your condition was discovered, your attitude about your diagnosis, and your outlook on life that makes a difference too. Your mindset is 100% under your control.

Gratitude changes your mental outlook. It can be a powerful tool for healing. Research indicates that gratitude is linked to improved mental strength, something critical for getting through your treatments. Gratitude also strengthens your immune system, lowers your blood pressure, staves off depression, increases your energy, and improves your sleep, all important factors for successful healing.

So, start and end your day be expressing gratitude. If you're religious, prayers are great, but if not simply say what you're grateful for, big or small, out loud. It makes a huge difference.

---

2 We've oversimplified this procedure for the sake of brevity, but the point is accurate. CAR-T isn't riskless, no cancer treatment is, but it has successfully been used to cure cancers like acute lymphoblastic leukemia, diffuse large B-cell lymphoma, follicular lymphoma, mantle cell lymphoma, and multiple myeloma.

*Scroll through
endless streams*

Information tides rise high

Seek the gems within

Google It, Maybe

You are going to want to research your illness. Know this, you are going to get the result that Google is forcing on you. This force, their algorithm, is based on your location, settings, query intent, user context, trending keywords, page quality, backlinks, etc., and is often populated by pharmaceutical ads, reviews, and other people's stories. It is not necessarily a bad thing, but it is a rabbit hole that can be less than helpful. We recommend you get the information you need and simultaneously do your best to avoid that proverbial rabbit hole.

Some of the more reputable online sources of cancer information include the American Cancer Society, The American Society of Clinical Oncology, The Mayo Clinic, The National Cancer Institute, and the Fred Hutchinson Cancer Research Center. See the website section of the bibliography for a more complete list.

There are over 200 different types of cancer, each with unique characteristics and treatments. Consequently, there are likely to be specialty organizations that focus on your condition, even if it's rare, such as The Myelodysplastic Syndromes Foundation, The Leukemia & Lymphoma Society, and Aplastic Anemia & MDS International Foundation who research and treat bone marrow and blood disorders, the National Breast Cancer Foundation, and the Prostate Cancer Foundation, among many others.

Be sure to assess the credibility of what you find by fact-checking information sources, leveraging multiple sites, and cross-referencing information. That seems like a lot of work, but this is about your health and well-being, so due diligence is worthwhile. There is good information out there, but also a lot of unhelpful garbage.

Once you understand the fundamentals of your situation, ask questions of your care team. It's not that different from learning a martial art. You're used to wading through the internet, balancing what you learn inside and outside of class, asking good questions, acquiring whatever is useful, and flushing the rest. You're doing the same thing with your medical condition.

Whispers in the heart
Silent prayers sent above
Faith's embrace, so warm

Lean Into Your Faith

Lawrence and Kris grew up with different religions, but are both people of faith, so there is a predisposition to prayer and an unwavering belief in God inherent in our makeup. If you are strong in your faith, lean in. If you are tepid in your faith, lean in. If you have fallen away, go back. If you have hesitancy because you don't want to be a hypocrite only seeking God when times are bad, don't be like that. What father would not welcome his child in their time of need?

While faith is no substitute for medical care, research indicates a strong connection between faith and healing. Studies by both Harvard University Medical School and the National Institutes of Health scientifically demonstrated this link, noting a positive effect of prayer on metabolism, heart rate, and blood pressure, among other things.

The relaxation response and the sense of self-efficacy gained through praying appears to strengthen the immune system. Although the role of religion played different roles in participants' lives, 85% of patients studied indicated that they used spirituality as a coping mechanism for dealing with illness and stress. It worked.

While it could be a placebo effect, it doesn't matter if it works, does it? Religious faith helps create a sense of purpose, hope, and meaning, all of which have profound psychological benefits such as reducing anxiety, stress, and depression. This improves mental health, strengthens coping mechanisms, and lets your body heal more effectively.

So, lean into your faith. It will help you get through your diagnosis, treatment, and recovery more easily.

Breath in stillness flows

Moments dance in
tranquil grace

Mindfulness takes root

Practice Mindfulness

Martial artists as a community tend to focus on things that we can influence or control while setting aside those things we cannot. You already know that. What you may not have considered is that this attitude is tremendously important for cancer patients and caregivers alike.

Mindfulness is the ability to be fully present in the moment, aware of where you are and what you're doing, yet not be overly reactive or overwhelmed by what is going on around you. Warrior ethos centers around this concept of living in the moment. Mindfulness is also at the root of Buddhism, Taoism, and many Native-American traditions, often applied through meditation or breathing exercises.

Life as a cancer patient can be stressful enough without compounding it by contemplating everything that can or could go wrong. Negative self-talk should have no place in your world. Mindful people can set aside things that are beyond their control, learn from the past, and plan for the future while living in the present. This attitude is scientifically proven to make a world of difference in stressful conditions like cancer diagnosis, treatment, and recovery.

When trying to calm yourself in stressful moments, you can focus on your breathing to regain control over your body. A common way to do that is often called "box-breathing." You may already be familiar with it from your training, but if you're not it works by breathing in through your nose and out through your mouth following a 4-count process.

Inhale for a 4-count, hold for a 4-count, exhale for a 4-count, and hold for a 4-count with empty lungs, all while concentrating on the act of breathing. It only takes a few minutes to achieve benefits from this technique. It's so powerful that it's taught not only to martial artists but also to elite operators in military and law enforcement too. In this fashion you can quickly break through the chaos, unclutter your mind, and achieve a state of purposeful focus.

Morning sun arises

Day begins with
clear intent

Ready hearts prevail

Buy More Underwear

Remember how we said you're going to throw up and told you to be ready for it? The same applies to your bowels. An explosion can happen unannounced. As much as you think you will be able to control it, you can't.

Do yourself a favor and buy more underwear so you can throw it away when accidents occur. Do not attempt to be frugal and wash your underwear. It's not worth the aggravation. Go get more underwear in preparation for accidents, they're going to happen. If you don't use them immediately, you will later. Even if we're wrong and you don't, you'll find a use for the underwear eventually.

Incidentally, TUCKS® medical cooling pads are a godsend when you find yourself using the bathroom multiple times a day. They help alleviate discomfort, burning, and itching, and can even shrink hemorrhoids that often pop up from over-frequent bowel movements, even if they're prolapsed. If you're chafing too, Aquaphor® works great.

Little things that improve your physical comfort can make a big difference in your mental outlook. Be prepared. Buy more underwear.

Maps and compass set
Journey waits on horizon
Prepared, we embark

Get to Know Your Staff

Walking down the hallway of the cancer treatment facility, Kris passed one of the receptionists.

"Have a good day, Kris."

"Thanks, Susan! You too."

As they continued down the hallway, Kris turned to his son Jackson, "I'm not sure being on a first-name basis with the receptionist at a cancer facility is a good thing."

Even though he hadn't recognized it at the time, the fact is that knowing your care team personally is a good thing. It's not just the doctors who are instrumental to your recovery. Receptionists, nurses, medical billers, patient navigators, case managers, and other support staff are key to moving through the treatment and recovery process with the least amount of friction.

You already have enough to deal with during your therapy, so anything that greases the wheels of the bureaucracy is a good thing. These folks can be helpful... or they can put in minimal effort. We are not implying that people in the medical profession would intentionally be unprofessional, however they are human. And, humans are emotional creatures.

In the same way, you get to know new students who come to the martial arts school where you train, you should get to know the staff at your medical facility too. As a patient you're just another number in the system. It's the people on your care team who turn you into a human; there's no downside to building good relationships with them.

Tempest in the soul

Unleashed in a
fierce outburst

Anger's brief control

You're Going to Get Short with People

You are going to get emotional with people. Think of your day as a bucket of emotion, in the morning it is full. As your day unfolds, the emotional bucket drains. Some days it drains rapidly, other days not so fast. When the emotional bucket gets to the bottom, you're drained. When you are drained you can become short, abrupt, or rude to others, especially those close to you, simply because they're in your proximity.

First, know this drain is inescapable. Your body is fighting. You have emotions and thoughts that can be dark, or at least challenging. Often these thoughts are kept internal to some degree, and these mental gymnastics draw on your emotional bucket.

Do your best to monitor your emotional bucket. Share the level of your mental container with those close to you, especially as it gets near the bottom. That will help you and help them. And, if you snap, become short or uncooperative, apologize. Your apology will be accepted 100% of the time.

The folks around you care about you. They know what you're going through. They want to help. And, they're human too. They might know that you didn't mean it, whatever that nasty thing was that you said, but it never hurts to apologize. Sure, you're going to get short with people from time-to-time, it's perfectly natural, but try not to be a dick about it.

Intricate design

Thread woven with
patient care

Tapestry unfolds

Do Her Socks Match?

You have a martial arts uniform. That uniform serves several purposes and so does the dress of your doctor. Kris' radiologist was a height and weight-appropriate, 40-year-old family man who wore slacks, dress shoes, and a well-starched dress shirt. Everything about the radiologist exuded precision. Combined with his pleasant personality, there was confidence in the forthcoming procedure.

The same thing goes for the nurse whose socks matched her shirt. The receptionist whose hair was in place and well done, it made him feel that he was working with professionals who would give him the highest level of care.

You're not wedded to your doctor. Lawrence went through three different oncologists before he found the physician he felt most comfortable with. Obviously, there's a lot more to being good at the job than dressing well, but it is an important indicator.

As a martial artist, if you tore your anterior cruciate ligament (ACL) would you rather go to a sports medicine doctor who looks like a professional bodybuilder or one who looks like a couch potato? Would you rather have a surgeon who pays attention to detail in all aspects of his or her appearance or take a risk with one who does not?

Lawrence's neighbor is a thoracic surgeon. His attention to detail is apparent in all aspects of his life, even in the fence he built between their houses, with grain-matching, perfectly stained, and spaced boards. Perfectionistic, perhaps, but exactly what you'd want in a surgeon. It didn't just look good; when a 50-foot-tall tree fell on it during a windstorm the fence barely suffered any damage because of how sturdily it had been built.

You might be the first to walk across the training floor and help a kid get their belt tied correctly. Being in order brings focus. As a martial artist, you know this. So, observe your healthcare professionals and how they dress. It is an outward expression of their focus. Attention to detail is important for good doctoring.

Dawn breaks

Sky ablaze, whispers
of promise arise

Fresh hopes fill the air

Each New Day Is a New Opportunity

Every day you wake up is a new opportunity. That day is a gift. If you opened a Christmas or birthday present and then threw it across the room, dismissing the gift, everyone around you would recoil, right? Think of each new morning in the same way. It might not be exactly what you were hoping for, but it's a gift nonetheless and should be appreciated.

Each day needs to be treated as a gift. What are you going to do with it? Yes, it can be hard, but you are built for this. Your training has given you the ability to find the gap, the moment of good.

There will be moments that are less than perfect. Recall the emotional bucket? When you wake up your bucket is full, and it allows you to set the tone for the day.

Are we suggesting it is easy? No. But, like we said, you are built for this. The more you train, the more you practice, the better you become. That applies to mindset just as much as it does to physical endeavors.

So, treat each new day as a new opportunity. It will improve your outlook. In fact, numerous scientific studies demonstrate that practicing gratitude just 15 minutes a day, five days a week reduces stress while improving your mood, relationships, quality of sleep, anxiety, pain levels, and longevity. And, more than 70 studies show a strong linkage between gratitude and mental health, such as lessening symptoms of depression.

Every day comes with new opportunity. Wake up, express gratitude, and embrace it.

Mountains touched
by clouds

Climbing paths
of excellence

Greatness at the peak

Finding a Great Doctor

Finding the right doctor is imperative. Your life is literally in their hands. You'll want someone who both understands your condition and who you feel comfortable working with. To complicate matters, in most instances, you will see a primary oncologist along with a variety of specialists, and you'll also be constrained by who your insurance provider(s) covers (or doesn't).

While you won't necessarily get to choose everyone on your care team, your primary oncologist is the most important, so let's focus on that. Referrals are great, and depending on how your diagnosis was discovered you may get one from your primary care physician, health maintenance organization, or friend or relative who's been in the same boat. Another option is MediFind (https://www.medifind.com/), a site that was created after the founder's brother was diagnosed with a semi-rare cancer and had trouble finding knowledgeable caregivers.

A hallmark of high intelligence is the ability to explain complex concepts in everyday language. If your doctor keeps throwing medical jargon your way, and you can't understand what they're talking about, that doesn't necessarily mean that they're stupid, they graduated medical school and passed their board exams after all, but it does mean that they're not the right provider for you. You'll need to understand diagnosis and treatment options well enough to make informed decisions. A good doctor will listen patiently, comfortably answer your concerns, and do it in a way that you can comprehend.

Your doctor should make you feel valued, not treated as a "number." Sure, you're talking with folks whose profession sees a lot of patients who don't recover so they can become jaded, but empathy and respect are important. You're not average and you shouldn't settle for an average doctor. You want a great one. Keep looking until you find someone who's a good fit. Here's a link to the American Cancer Society's checklist on how to choose a good doctor: https://www. cancer.org/content/dam/cancer-org/cancer-control/en/worksheets/ choosing-a-doctor-worksheet.pdf.

Black and white entwine
Yin and yang in harmony
Details balance light

If You're Burned on the Outside, You're Burned on the Inside

It seems obvious, but it is not often said regarding radiation treatments: They will burn you. You will likely have some skin peeling, like a sunburn. That's what you see on the outside, but you are also burned on the inside of your body.

That is the goal of radiation treatment, to burn the cancer cells, killing or shrinking them, while minimizing damage to healthy surrounding tissue. As the radiation treatment progresses over time both outside and inside burns will take place, and you need to be prepared for that. It's not that the radiologist hasn't explained this phenomenon, but sometimes in the hailstorm of information, that idea can get lost.

Radiation is a common treatment for many types of cancer, including tumors on the head, neck, breast, lung, and prostate. There are two major types, external beam therapy where radiation is directed from outside the body, and internal radiation therapy where radioactive substances are implanted near the tumor. Side effects can include skin redness, irritation, burns, fatigue, nausea, and hair loss, among other things.

The trauma of radiation therapy can be remediated to some degree when you eat a nutritious diet and stay hydrated. Choose real food, avoiding anything with ingredients you can't pronounce to the extent feasible. Hydrate more than you think you need to and consider adding water-rich foods like cucumber, berries, and watermelon to your diet.

Skincare matters too. Consult with your care team, but generally speaking, you'll want to use mild, fragrance-free soaps, apply moisturizers, and protect treatment areas from direct sunlight. They might suggest loose-fitting, natural fiber clothing too as that's better tolerated than synthetics by many patients.

Wisdom softly speaks

*Guiding light in
times of doubt*

Paths unfold with ease

You're Going to Get a Lot of Advice

If you tell people about your condition, you are going to get advice from every direction. It may be a person who has gone through treatment and succeeded. It may come in the form of a story about a friend, colleague, or second cousin. You may receive emails with articles attached about some new promising treatment that may or may not apply to your unique situation.

Every one of these interactions comes from love. They care. Don't dismiss the information or the stories for two reasons: The first reason is you may find a nugget of information upon which you can take action. What are we but action-oriented? You didn't get that belt you earned by sitting on the couch. Secondly, these stories and information will serve as a pick-me-up, a boost to your attitude. And you know what? You are going to take every boost you can, no matter how big or small.

It probably goes without saying, but don't take action on these suggestions without talking to your care team first. Sometimes you'll need to reconcile different opinions among specialists, but general advice may or may not apply to your individual condition and treatment regimen. Seek to educate yourself to the maximum extent feasible. After all, you're your own best advocate, but it's really hard to advocate intelligently without education.

Be sure to thank everyone for their advice, even if you're unable to use it. It shows how much they care.

Morning light breaks clear

Plans laid out, tools
at the ready

Day's task set with care

When You Think You Will Not Need the Paperwork Again, You Will

Keep every piece of paperwork, every .pdf, form, and file. Order it and put it in a place where you can access it. You will need that information many times over. This small amount of quality control will save you hours of frustration. When we say every piece of information, we mean it. The medical system is a complicated maze of repetition, replication, and redundancy. In other words, it's a bureaucracy.

You will be impressed with some aspects of communication within the system. You will also be stunned that some departments don't communicate well. It's up to you to be prepared. No one advocates better for you than you.

According to a Harvard University study, half of U.S. cancer patients experience problems with coordination of care, including receiving conflicting information from various providers and insurance agencies. As a result of delays, denials, and deductibles, many patients use most or all of their savings or go into debt during their treatment despite having insurance.

You will likely be dealing with your healthcare provider and insurance agency directly, but this becomes exponentially more complicated when you coordinate care across multiple specialists. The good news is that there are experts who can help you navigate the system and agencies that help with transportation, caregiver expenses, short-term housing during treatment, and supplemental or disability income replacement if you can't work during treatments. In other words, there's a lot of help out there.

Cancer is expensive to treat and both procedures and medical payments may be delayed or denied if the paperwork isn't done just right, such as when incorrect or outdated billing codes are used. Oftentimes once you think everything has wrapped up successfully, it will be retroactively scrutinized by an audit after the fact. So, expect that if it can go wrong, it will, and keep records of everything to help straighten things out as quickly as possible afterward.

Stars light the night sky

Dreams weave
through quiet mind

Rest in tranquil arms

Sleep On It

The old saying, "I'm going to sleep on it," is a statement of physical and psychological truth. When things are not going well, especially at the end of the day when your emotional bucket is drained, sleep on it. For optimal health, adults need roughly 7 to 9 hours of sleep a night, more if you're recovering from surgery or certain therapies. A good night's sleep helps lower your blood pressure, relax and repair your muscles, regulate your body temperature, rejuvenate your skin, and boost your infection-fighting T-cells, among a host of other health benefits.

So yes, go to bed. Let your body rest. Let your brain clear out the sludge. Certainly, "sludge" is not a technical term, but studies have shown your brain needs sleep to remove accumulated proteins. One of the proteins that is flushed out on a nightly basis is beta-amyloid. The accumulation of this protein in your brain is considered a hallmark of Alzheimer's disease, and deep rapid eye movement (REM) sleep helps protect against beta-amyloid buildup. We include beta-amyloid as a proof-point of science validating the old adage of sleeping on it.

Problems won't often disappear overnight, yet your ability to handle them increases with a good night's sleep. Whenever it seems overwhelming, meditate, focusing on your breathing to clear your mind just like you learned in martial arts. That will help you fall sleep quicker and slumber more restfully.

As if you don't have enough to deal with already, many cancer patients suffer from insomnia. If meditation and breathing isn't sufficient to calm your mind and help you drift off, a pharmaceutical-grade melatonin supplement, such as those prescribed by a naturopathic doctor, will usually do the trick. Check with your care team.

Good sleep benefits both your mental and physical health, including enhancing metabolism, immune function, creativity, cognitive function, focus, and concentration. So, if you're having a tough time, sleep on it.

In a moment's glance

Stories unfold,
worlds collide

Seeing with deep care

The Baader-Meinhof Phenomenon

The Baader-Meinhof phenomenon is often called the Frequency Illusion. It works this way: If you purchase a new car, you rapidly begin to see the brand and model you purchased on every road you drive. There aren't any more of them out there than there were yesterday, well perhaps the one you're driving, but suddenly you're perceiving them more frequently because your brain is focused on the pattern. You placed that pattern in your own mind with the purchase of your new vehicle. This is a good thing if you use it to your advantage.

The Frequency Illusion served us well as hunter-gatherers in the ancient past, such as with the ability to recognize edible berries versus poisonous ones. We are biologically built for pattern recognition. It's a product of our evolution. Pattern recognition isn't inherently good or bad in the modern world, it's what we do with it that matters.

Simply put, focus on the bad and you will find the bad. Focus on the good and you will find the good. It is all about tuning your mind. As a cancer patient, building and using the Frequency Illusion to your advantage is essential. It keeps you from spiraling into darkness. And, you will find that as a martial artist, tuning your mind will not take long.

What do we do as martial artists other than repetitions? That's how we learn the fundamentals, climb through the ranks, and strive to master our style. Leveraging the Baader-Meinhof phenomenon is no different. After a few repetitions, you will find the handle and at that point you can make the technique your own.

Use the Baader-Meinhof phenomenon and use it well. Focus on the positive. It will change your outlook for the better which is tremendously important to assure the best outcome from your treatment regimen.

Sunrise paints the sky
Joy in every waking breath
Day's potential blooms

No Bad Days

Often you will hear people say, "I'm having a bad day." You can expect to hear this from pretty much everyone around you—friends, coworkers, neighbors, and family members. This statement condemns the day to failure and darkens every experience from the moment it's uttered, in part because of the aforementioned Baader-Meinhof effect.

This phrase, "I'm having a bad day," often comes from a psychological phenomenon called "catastrophizing," a mental habit of anticipating the worst possible outcome in any given situation, even when it is highly unlikely. Catastrophizing is a distortion. It is a situation where a person assumes the worst rather than pragmatically assessing what's truly going on. Catastrophizing is a negative dance of the mind. It is full of exaggeration, drama, and negative outcomes.

If you are dancing this dance, know what is leading the dance. It's not you. Look at the thought, the negative assumption, and challenge it. Here is a perspective that can aid you in making the mental shift and challenging those negative thoughts: There are no bad days, only fleeting bad moments.

If you are throwing up from radiation therapy, it is only a moment. Afterward, you will feel a little better. Dreading the day of radiation therapy is not productive, it creates anxiety and bolsters fear. These emotions have no use for you. It is only a moment in time, not the entirety of your day. Even on your worst day, there will be moments of good, just like on your best day some tiny bad thing might occur.

There are bad moments, not bad days. Remember that.

Predator's sharp gaze
Hunted in the silent night
Fear in shadows' depth

Threats And Blackmail

Martial artists by nature tend to be a stoic group. When faced with adversity chances are good that you often choose to shoulder the burden alone rather than asking others for help. Sometimes, however, the choice of whether or not to be forthcoming about your condition falls outside of your control.

For example, if you have to miss a significant amount of work or school for inpatient treatments, you'll have to say something when asking for leave. In this illustration you can limit disclosure to a small circle of folks who know what's going on and will keep it in confidence if you want them to, but in other instances that becomes impossible.

In 2023, some 800,000 cancer patients in the United States discovered that their name, Social Security Number, home address, phone number, medical history, lab test results, and insurance information were compromised by a data breach at the Fred Hutchinson Cancer Research Center. Shortly thereafter, many were contacted by hackers who threatened to leak their personal information if they didn't pay up.

Sadly, this type of blackmail isn't uncommon. According to Cybersecurity Ventures, cybercriminals wrested about $1.1B dollars from their victims in 2023, and that's only the ones who paid. Battling cancer is a challenge, extortion makes it worse.

You should know that cancer patients in the U.S. have legal protections under a variety of laws including the Health Insurance Portability and Accountability Act (HIPPA), the Americans with Disabilities Act (ADA), and the Family and Medical Leave Act (FMLA), to name a few. That doesn't remediate having to deal with identity theft or other hassles if your information is stolen, but it does mean that if your diagnosis gets out more publicly than you'd like you have certain protections under the law. You can take legal action if you want to. Further, if your employer treats you unfairly because of your condition, the U.S. Equal Employment Opportunity Commission (EEOC) will help you.

Seeds planted with care

*Harvest reaps the
labor's fruit*

Effort's sweet reward

Consider Clinical Trials

Clinical trials are studies of new treatments, or novel uses of existing therapies, on patients who volunteer to undergo them. These experiments can be risky, but can also create opportunities for you because if you're accepted you will get access to cutting-edge treatments that are not available to the general public, typically at little or no cost.

By participating in a clinical trial, you can help contribute to medical research designed to create better outcomes for cancer patients in the future. This requires informed consent so you'll understand the risks and opportunities that you're signing up for and go in eyes wide open.

Volunteers must meet strict criteria appropriate for each study. To assure patient safety to the extent feasible, studies are monitored by internal review boards, data safety monitoring boards, clinical investigators, and federal agencies such as the Office for Human Research Protections (OHRP), the National Cancer Institute (NCI), and the Food and Drug Administration (FDA).

There are four phases of clinical trials that you might become involved with, three of which must be completed before submitting new treatments to the FDA for approval in most instances. Phase I studies identify the highest safe dose that can be given to patients without causing severe side effects. Phase II trials ascertain whether or not the treatment works on certain types of cancer. Phase III trials compare the safety and effectiveness of the new treatment against current standard treatments. Once approved, new treatments are often observed over a long period in phase IV studies to assure ongoing safety and better understand how they impact patient quality of life over time.

You may be notified about relevant clinical trials by someone on your care team who can help you decide whether or not a study is a good option for you. Alternatively, you can proactively search for applicable studies at the National Cancer Institute, Center for Information and Study on Clinical Research Participation, or EmergingMed Clinical Trial Navigation Service. Their websites are listed in the bibliography.

Steps toward the dawn

Future calls with
bright promise

Forward we advance

Keep 'Er Movin'

This statement, "keep 'er movin'," is a Midwestern maxim. The Midwest of America is generally known as a place of common sense, straight-ahead application, and neighborly behavior. Unlike what's common along certain portions of the East and West coasts, strangers in the elevator say "hi" in the Midwest, folks there hold the door open for you. All of these are wonderful attributes.

Keep 'er movin' is a simple encouragement said to another person when moments become complicated, or direction is lost. Two farmhands are not focusing on their job at the moment, doing something potentially unsafe, the boss may say, "Keep 'er movin'." The kids are not getting out the door for the school play or football practice fast enough, "Keep 'er movin'." You get the idea…

We love this gentle admonishment to re-focus and get to the task at hand. We recommend you internalize this phrase and lean into it when needed. It is simple, direct, and enhancing.

You see, when you're moving you are getting things done, not dwelling on extraneous things that inhibit your progress. And, as you know from progressing through the ranks of your martial arts system, big or small, accomplishments add up. This creates a habit of success, which in turn breeds more success. It's a positive, self-sustaining cycle.

The wonderful part of internalizing this Midwestern maxim is that it works, and it works instantly. So, keep 'er movin'.

Wounds reveal the truth

Scarlet drops on
pale canvas

Blood tells silent tales

You Will Bleed

Bleeding is a common problem for cancer patients. If the cancer itself doesn't decrease your platelet[3] counts enough to increase bleeding and bruising risks, the treatment regimen just might. Chemotherapy, radiation, anti-inflammatory drugs, anticoagulants, and the like can cause catastrophic bleeding, episodic major bleeding, or low-volume oozing, and can manifest as incidents like nosebleeds, gum bleeds, vomiting blood, blood in your urine or stool, small red spots on your skin that cluster together like a rash, excessive bleeding from small nicks or cuts, fever, fatigue, or unexplained bruising.

Check with your care team before taking any anti-inflammatory supplements, using over-the-counter medications that can increase bleeding like aspirin, ibuprofen, or naproxen, or having elective surgery or any type dental work done. To further reduce your risk, switch from a bladed razor to electric if you shave, use soft-bristled toothbrushes, switch from traditional dental floss to a water flosser, and be extra careful when using sharp instruments. It's generally a good idea to avoid walking around barefoot too.

Learn basic first aid, stock up on bandages, gauze pads, medical tape, and antibiotic ointment, and keep a first aid kit handy at all times, including in your vehicle. If your platelet counts are very low, or you're prone to accidents, it may be a good idea to buy a hemostatic agent like QuikClot®, Woundstat™, or Celox™. They were designed for treating major injuries like gunshots and stab wounds, hence can quickly stop bleeding, but can also cause thermal tissue injury when used, so check with your care team.

If your bleeding is severe, won't stop after 15 minutes of direct pressure, requires use of a hemostatic agent, or is accompanied by dizziness, fainting, or shock, seek medical attention immediately. If you get a lot of nosebleeds, vasoconstricting nasal sprays like Afrin® can make them stop more easily. For minor gum bleeding, the tannins in black tea can help, just press a teabag against your gums for a bit.

---

3 Platelets are small, colorless cell fragments that travel throughout your bloodstream. When blood vessels are damaged, platelets aggregate together (coagulate) at the site of the injury to prevent excessive bleeding.

Colors softly mix

Canvas breathes
with shades of life

Blending hues unite

The Holidays Will Blur

Your birthday, and other days of importance, holidays, graduations, weddings, and the like, they will all blur. It is hard to find energy these days. The thermonuclear blast of your battle obfuscates and dominates your days. It can be hard to find the specialness of these distinctive moments after your diagnosis, especially on treatment days if you're experiencing chemotherapy, radiation, or other physically and mentally challenging therapies.

In the same way that your martial arts instructor encourages you to do your best, we suggest you do the same with these special days and moments. Your 100% that you are accustomed to giving on these days may fall short of what you would normally have expected from yourself. It may be a challenge, and you may want to opt out, but we suggest giving that 100% anyway. Here's why: These moments are not only special, but normal.

You may not have thought of it this way, but you crave normalcy. Any place where you can find it, do it. Normal is good.

Try reframing things this way: If your current head-space is that you are falling short in your participation based on what you used to be able to do, we assure you that you're not. You are giving your best under the conditions you face now, today. That's what matters most.

It is a balancing act that may require a nap in the afternoon to have the energy you need for the coming event that night. You may need somebody to drive you, or you may need take your medications early in preparation. Whatever you need, make the effort, set yourself up for success, and participate. Never check out on the special days, the special moments.

You crave normalcy and now it is not normal time. But you can meet the moment and seize that time. With a little preparation you can elevate the important moments that highlight life and keep them from becoming a homogenous blur.

In the artisan's hands

Swordsmith's fire
brings life to steel

Mastery in craft

Sliced, Diced, Poked and Prodded

I met this distinguished gentleman. He took me back to his place, made me feel comfortable, then gave me a roofie. And then, as the sedative kicked in, he cut me. He was a great doctor. I can barely even see the scar today.

You can expect to be sliced, diced, poked, and prodded. Depending on what type of cancer you're being treated for there will be blood tests, biopsies, surgeries, chemo ports, intravenous line infusions, and various other invasive procedures. That's not normal, or at least it didn't used to be.

Let's face it, most folks don't love the thought of foreign objects being shoved into their bodies repeatedly, but nowadays that's your situation. One way to get through it all more easily is through meditation.

If you've been studying a classical martial art, you likely begin and end class with meditation, so you already know this. You don't have to use the *seiza* (kneeling) posture from class, you can sit or lie down in any comfortable position. Close your eyes and focus on your breathing, using the four-count, box-breathing we described earlier.

As you begin to relax, pick a point of your body, drawing your focus to that part. Oftentimes it's easier to start from your feet and move up, but you could just as easily start with your head and move down. Regardless, pick one point at a time, say the big toe on your right foot or the heel of your left foot. Be mindful of any sensations in this area, including any pain or discomfort. If it hurts, acknowledge that and any associated emotions while continuing your box-breathing. By observing the discomfort, you aren't likely to alleviate it all that much, but you can help your body relax and accept it.

Once you've finished, slowly shift your focus to the next body part and the next, until you've covered your whole body one small part at a time. It may take 30 to 45 minutes or so, but by the time you're done, you'll find that you are able to disassociate the pain and fear, using mindfulness to control your body. The more you do this the easier it is to reduce the stress of your treatments.

Curiosity

Questions spark the quest for truth

Knowledge blossoms bright

Know Your Nurses

Your nurses have seen it all. They have their sleeves rolled up and are in the fray. You need to lean into them. They are not going to give medical advice, that's for doctors, but they do have tips and tricks that make a big difference. "If you tape that feeding tube to your chest up here you will get better results and the tube won't bother you when you are sleeping."

Many nurses are masters of emotions too. That is to say they have seen your situation before, the emotional and the physical, and understand what you're going through. They aren't clergy, but can connect you with them if you so desire, "Would you like a priest, pastor, imam, or rabbi to pray with you before your surgery?"

And they have skills at the psychological level too. As an example, Kris was going in for a biopsy, not a complicated procedure, with only local anesthesia needed. Somehow, some way, the moment started to escalate emotionally as he lay on the gurney. Was it a lack of sleep that initiated the escalation? Could it have been the unusual and unknown environment? Was it a combination of those and or other unknown factors? Hard to say, but he felt himself begin to spiral.

Kris turned to his nurse and said, "I'm not doing very well, and I don't know why."

The nurse, a man of about 40 years of age, replied, "What's going on?"

They talked for a bit and the nurse used his skills to get to the heart of the matter. He sensed that Kris needed more information about the procedure and provided it. All Kris knew before that point was that he was having a biopsy and what time to report to the hospital, so the additional information was illuminating. The nurse ended the conversation with, "I'll be with you during and after as well." That made all the difference.

Everyone on your care team plays a role. Nurses are multidimensional professionals. Lean into what they have to offer; it can knock the rough edges off your world.

Seeds cast to the wind

Nature's gamble
in the breeze

Chances bloom and grow

Never Tell Me the Odds

There's a famous quote from Han Solo, a smuggler played by actor Harrison Ford in the Star Wars™ movie *The Empire Strikes Back,* "Never tell me the odds." In that scene, he was navigating an asteroid field in a small spaceship, a situation where most pilots would have crashed into something and died. His quip was in response to another character, the droid C-3PO played by actor Anthony Daniels, saying, "Sir, the possibility of successfully navigating an asteroid field is approximately 3,720 to 1."

While entertaining, Star Wars isn't real. But Solo's point is well taken for your situation nonetheless. The American Cancer Society (ACS) tracks 5-year survival rates for 22 types of cancer, with averages ranging from a high of 100% to a low of 36%. Odds change for the worse if your cancer was caught in a later stage or has metastasized.

Sure, this is a source of data, a useful one, but don't overfocus on these statistics. The data tends to be short- to mid-term, not long-term, so you're not seeing the whole picture. More importantly, never forget that others with your condition are normal and you're not. You're not that typical, average, median-model person who fits the statistic exactly. You're a martial artist.

Sitting in the waiting room where 37 other individuals had queued up to get their blood tests at Virginia Mason Medical Center, Lawrence was surprised to note that he was the only person in the crowd, a majority of whom looked younger than him, who wasn't overweight. Most folks who develop cancer have risk factors beforehand such as obesity, excessive alcohol use, smoking, poor diet, chronic inflammation, or other considerations that are rare in martial artists. Mentally and physically we're simply not average.

Sure, there might be some genetic cause of your condition too, but our point is that as a martial artist, you stand out from the crowd. You're an outlier, not the mean. Don't think that the odds apply to you. They might, but chances are good that they won't.

Savory delight

Flavors dance on
eager tongues

Feast of pure joy shared

Intermittent Fasting

Numerous scientific studies demonstrate that intermittent fasting, such as eating during a 6-hour window and fasting for the remaining 18 hours of your day, can trigger a metabolic switch that goes from glucose-based to ketone-based energy. This physiological effect improves heart health, physical performance, working memory, stress resistance, and longevity while decreasing the incidence of several diseases, including type 2 diabetes, neurodegenerative disorders, inflammatory bowel disease, and several varieties of cancer.

It makes logical sense that intermittent fasting is beneficial. After all, before our ancestors learned how to band together, build communities, and farm the land, they were hunter-gatherers. It took a lot of energy to find food each day, and some days were unproductive, so our bodies were genetically designed to thrive for long periods of time without eating.

With today's sedentary lifestyles, overeating is a challenge. In fact, according to the CDC's National Center for Health Statistics (NCHS), 40.3% of adults were obese in the United States as of August of 2023, a factor that's directly linked to 13 different types of cancer. It's hard to control your caloric intake if you have multiple meals and snacks throughout the day. If, on the other hand, you condense your intake into a small number of healthy, fulfilling meals, you can more easily satisfy your nutritional needs and feel full without overeating.

Since most folks have trouble sleeping soundly when they're hungry, shifting the eating window later in your day makes it easier to eat what you like without "cheating." So, consider skipping breakfast while consuming zero-calorie beverages like black coffee, green tea, and water, and waiting until early afternoon before you eat anything. Once you start, stop eating within six hours.

There's value in intermittent fasting, but it's not for everyone, especially if you're using a feeding tube, having trouble eating enough calories, or have difficulty keeping food down. Check with your care team to see if it is right for you.

Falsehood's fragile mask

Cracks appear in
guilty light

Lies unravel slow

Beware of Scam "Cures"

In December of 1979, actor Steve McQueen (1930 – 1980) was diagnosed with pleural mesothelioma, a type of lung cancer, likely caused by asbestos exposure from when he served in the United States Marine Corps. His doctors tried chemotherapy and radiation, but quickly discovered that wasn't working, stopped treatments, and told him to make good use of what little time he had left. As you can imagine, Steve McQueen was a U.S. Marine, he refused to give up.

In his search for a cure, McQueen found Dr. William Donald Kelley (1905 – 2005), a dentist who claimed he could cure cancer through natural healing. Kelley's clinic was located in Mexico because he had lost his license to practice in the United States. He treated McQueen with coffee enemas, shampooing, and a variety of vitamins and minerals, along with laetrile, a drug made from apricot pits which was determined to be both unsafe and ineffective by the FDA. Laetrile is illegal in the U.S. today.

Desperate people do desperate things, and unfortunately, that makes cancer patients an easy target for misinformation. There are more than 200 different types of cancer, and no treatment that works for everything, so stay away from so-called universal cures. There aren't any. Further, "natural" doesn't necessarily mean safe. Some of the deadliest toxins known to man, cyanide, abrin, and botulinum, are all-natural substances.

Because the scientific method is related to testing and disproving hypotheses, scientists tend to use soft words like "correlate," "support," or "associated" rather than hard words like "proven," "conclusive," or "definitive." This nomenclature can be a clue that what you're reading is suspect. Further, supplements and complementary medications can cause adverse interactions with your conventional therapy.

Casting a broad net is good, just exercise caution while doing it. Do your homework and consult with your care team before trying anything new. Here's a short video about avoiding cancer scams that can help: https://www.cancer.gov/about-cancer/managing-care/using-trusted-resources/health-info-online.

Falling meteor

Sky's gift lands
with fiery crash

Earth forever marked

Dealing With Shock

In the front row of health class, a young man went rigid. He was in shock. The film on open-heart surgery hit him hard. The instructor, having seen that reaction before, stepped forward and gently brought the student back. After the crisis was settled, he explained that shock can be unpredictable, sometimes ignited by something as simple as a blood draw or instructional video.

There are multiple kinds of shock. Hypovolemic shock comes from blood loss, whereas cardiogenic shock occurs when the heart is unable to pump enough blood to meet the body's needs. There's a low likelihood that you will experience either of these.

Disruptive shock includes septic (severe infections), anaphylactic (allergic reactions), neurogenic (blood pooling in your extremities), and obstructive (blocked blood vessels). Once again, while it could happen, you're unlikely to have to deal with any of these during your treatment and if you do there's likely to be a medical professional there to take care of you.

Emotional or psychological shock, on the other hand, is fairly common in cancer patients. It stems from an intense response to traumatic events. As you go through your diagnosis, treatment, and recovery process, know that shock can show-up from multiple sources and with varying intensity. It is not a sign of weakness, it's quite commonplace. Your task is to be aware of what your body is doing and take action when necessary.

If you feel anxiety, fear, physical numbness, disassociation, disbelief, confusion, or similar feelings of becoming overwhelmed, recognize that you could be in shock. The first step is to make your body safe by lying down and focusing on your breathing. Breathe slowly and deeply, loosening any restrictive clothing as necessary to do so. Elevate your feet above the level of your heart. A blanket covering your core will help too.

Once you have your body back under control, you can audit the triggering event to figure out what happened. It may be advisable to reach out to a mental health professional too.

Eyes seek the unknown
Curiosity's deep well
Questions spark new paths

Don't Be Afraid to Ask

The process of cancer diagnosis, treatment, and rehabilitation is complex. There are often two types of medicine at play, conventional medicine performed by doctors who treat you with drugs, radiation, or surgery, and integrative medicine performed by doctors who address biological (e.g., diet, supplementation), mind-body (e.g., acupuncture. meditation, biofeedback), or manipulative (e.g., massage, chiropractic, reflexology) treatments that can complement the conventional cures to help remediate side effects and speed healing.

It takes a team of healthcare providers and support personnel to get you through. Your team will likely include medical oncologists (doctors who specialize in cancer care), surgical oncologists (who specialize in cancer surgery), radiologists (who administer radiation treatments), oncology nurses (who provide supporting care), patient navigators (who help you navigate the healthcare system), psychologists (who help with your mental health), social workers (who specialize in emotional support, counseling, and referrals), rehabilitation therapists (who help restore function after treatments), dieticians (who help with your nutritional needs), home health aides (who help with daily chores), clergy (who provide spiritual guidance), and pharmacists (who fulfill your prescriptions), to name the primary players.

That's a pretty big group, and they don't always communicate with each other effectively. Consequently, it's important that you play point guard, to use a sports analogy. Point guards in basketball are responsible for controlling the ball, setting up plays for success, and initiating the offense. When it comes to cancer, that pretty much sums up your job description. You're on point; your medical team is all about helping you succeed.

Ask questions about your proposed treatment regimen, its benefits, risks, and side effects. Ask about what happens before, during, and after your therapy. Understand any relevant clinical trials. Seek second and third opinions, and do your best to reconcile different perspectives amongst practitioners. The only stupid question is the one you don't ask. So, keep asking until you feel comfortable with your knowledge.

Steady hands persist

Routine carves
strength in silence

Discipline's calm force

Staying in Shape

Learning martial arts can be challenging. For many practitioners it's a lifelong process, one that encompasses not only internalizing an abundance of physical techniques and mental disciplines, but also learning new methods of body alignment, breathing, and movement. As you know, diligent practice builds the physical strength, endurance, and flexibility necessary to progress amongst the ranks. You've worked hard to achieve your status, no matter how high or low it currently is, and you won't let anything, even cancer, derail your progress.

Research shows that for most people with cancer, exercise is safe and beneficial. Unless your care team says otherwise, you can and should continue physical activity before, during, and after your treatments. If you become inactive overlong you risk muscle weakness, reduced range of motion, and loss of body function.

Regular exercise helps your body and brain work better, strengthens your immune system, helps you maintain a healthy weight, and improves your overall quality of life. Exercise simultaneously reduces some treatment side effects like fatigue, depression, and anxiety, and even decreases the chances of certain types of cancers reoccurring after you complete your therapy.

Work with your care team to determine what you can and cannot safely do. Generally, you'll want to start slow and build up, focusing on stretching and movement first before continuing on to more vigorous exercise like aerobics, resistance training, weightlifting, or martial arts, but the better shape you're in before you start cancer treatments, the more you'll likely be able to do during your therapy. You're already an athlete.

Even if you're not feeling up to lifting weights or other intensive "workouts," you can usually maintain or increase your non-exercise activity thermogenesis through walking your dog, gardening, playing with your kids, washing your car, or even simple things like using a standing desk. Our point, you were in good shape before your diagnosis, don't stop exercising after. It's good for you.

Voices rise in strength

Claiming rights and
making change

Agency's bold stand

Right to Try

If your condition is diagnosed early enough most cancers are treatable, yet all malignancies aren't the same. There are some varieties that doctors and scientists know very little about. Cancers are considered rare when they affect less than 40,000 people per year in the United States. By way of comparison, there were 313,510 new incidents of breast cancer, 299,010 of prostate cancer, 234,580 of lung cancer, and 152,810 cases of colorectal cancer diagnosed in the United States in 2024.

Some cancers are extremely rare. For example, Lawrence's uncle passed away from appendiceal cancer, a condition that affected fewer than 1,500 people a year at the time. These unusual cancers don't get the same level of investment and research that more common varieties do, hence often have less treatment options and lower recovery rates.

In 2017 congress passed the "Right to Try Act" and it became law in 2018. This act allows patients with life-threatening conditions like cancer to access experimental treatments that haven't been approved by the FDA yet. The philosophy behind this law was that if standard options have been exhausted and clinical trials are not available for them, patients should have the right to opt for longshot cures after consultation with their care team. These investigational treatments must have completed Phase I clinical trials, but not have been approved or licensed by the FDA in order to be eligible.

If you have a rare condition, or a more common one where your treatment regimen isn't working, and you're are interested in pursuing this alternative, you should discuss options with your doctor. Companies who develop investigational treatments can provide information to your care team about whether or not their drug or biologic product is eligible under the Right to Try Act. If so, your doctor can help you determine whether the opportunity is worth the risk.

Because these treatments have not been proven safe or effective yet, they come with higher risk than common treatments or later-phase clinical trials. Nevertheless, if you're running out of options, participating could be your best shot.

In a fleeting glance

Stories hidden
deep revealed

Seeing with clear eyes

Negativity Bias

Remember a time when you made special plans, say taking someone you care about to a nice restaurant or show. You were excited. You made reservations and planned the whole night in detail. You dressed up, arrived early, and had a great time only to return to your vehicle to find a parking ticket. Suddenly all you could think about was the citation. That's an example of the negativity effect.

This negative bias, or negativity effect, is a psychological preconception that causes you to focus on the negative, even when positive or neutral things of equal or greater intensity occur. That means that unpleasant or harmful memories, thoughts, emotions, and interactions can stand out more than pleasant ones. That's not a good thing, and it affects your mood, the way you evaluate the world around you, and how you make decisions.

Generally speaking, cancer isn't a good thing either, we'd much rather not have it, but it's not all bad. It reframes what's important to you. It improves your appreciation of life, friends, family, and relationships, often helping you bond better with your loved ones. It shows you who your friends truly are. And, it can be a powerful force for personal growth. But you have to get past the negativity effect in order to find the positive in your circumstances.

Practicing mindfulness and cultivating gratitude can help you move past the negativity bias, reframing what's going on in your life for the better. Notice your harmful thoughts and understand how they affect your emotions and behaviors. Confront them logically and dispassionately. Oftentimes it helps to write things down. Armed with this perspective you can begin to alter your internal dialogue. As with anything else, it gets easier with practice.

If you find yourself spiraling hard, don't hesitate to reach out to a professional counselor, psychiatrist, social worker, or spiritual guide. You don't have to go through this alone.

Chest swells with
bright strength

Accomplishments
gleam like gold

Pride's firm stance upheld

Stand Up

Cancer treatment can be exhausting. This exhaustion can manifest in many ways such as unhealthy skin pallor and unwanted weight loss. It can also affect your posture, oftentimes without you even realizing it.

We suggest that no matter how you feel, you should make a deliberate effort to stand up straight and walk with purpose. If you don't feel like it, do your best. If you think you are performing for others when you stand up and walk with purpose, you are. More importantly, you are performing for yourself.

You may be surprised to know that a Harvard University Medical School study discovered that good posture can improve your mood. For example, patients who sat up straight improved their symptoms of anxiety, stress, and depression. The same phenomena applies when you're moving too. Good posture can increase your positive thoughts, improve memory, and aid recall, increasing your dopamine and testosterone levels while reducing cortisol[4].

By standing up and walking with purpose you are using your body to help your emotional state. When you catch yourself slouching, straighten your spine. If you are shuffling, straighten your spine and walk heel to toe. The more you do this the more your positive body position flows.

As a small addition, Kris opens every door he can for others too. It is of course a courtesy, but it is also an act of self-value.

---

4 Cortisol is an adrenal hormone that's linked to stress. It helps you get through danger, but too much of it over a long period of time is harmful. It can increase blood pressure, suppress your immune system, and cause gastrointestinal issues like ulcers, among other things.

Billowing giants

Heaven's canvas
gently swirls

Clouds paint
fleeting dreams

Anesthesia And Brain-Fog

Depending on what drugs are used, anesthesia generally clears out of your system within 24 hours, yet the effects of the sedatives can linger in your body for up to thirty days, more or less. Anesthesia can create brain-fog, known as postoperative cognitive dysfunction. That's a fancy way of saying that you are likely to discover after surgery that you lack the clarity to which you have become accustomed, at least for a while. It's not uncommon to "lose" a day or more in the process.

As the anesthesia wears off its important to focus on getting adequate rest, staying hydrated, eating well, managing pain, and engaging in mental activities that can re-stimulate your brain while you're recovering from the surgery. Acupuncture has been shown to help too.

One way we've found to accelerate the brain-clearing process is through exercise. We are not going to suggest what form of exercise you choose other than to say that some of it is better than none. Do as much as you can, whatever your care team clears you to do.

And finally, give yourself a break if you are temporarily not as mentally fast as you once were. Take a pause, clear your thoughts, and re-que your questions or responses to other people's questions. You are okay. The lethargy isn't you; it's the drugs. They'll wear off soon.

Laughter's healing touch

Eases burdens,
lifts the soul

Magic in each smile

Laughter Is (kinda) The Best Medicine

Cancer is no laughing matter, but in some ways it should be. Scientific evidence demonstrates that a good laugh has both short- and long-term health benefits. When you laugh it doesn't just release endorphins that can improve your mental perspective, it causes physical changes in your body too.

A good laugh quickly increases the supply of oxygen to your body, stimulating your heart, brain, lungs, and muscles. Over time, positive thoughts release neuropeptides that help you fight stress which, in turn, can improve your immune system. That's why laughing on a regular basis can lessen the impact of anxiety and depression, improving your mood, increasing your ability to cope with difficult situations, strengthening your heart, and (to some degree) even relieving everyday aches and pains.

A good sense of humor can strengthen your relationships too, helping you get along better with others, defuse conflict, and bond more deeply. There's no downside to that. While laughter is great, even a simple smile is good. Forcing yourself to smile, even when you're faking it, can lighten your mood by releasing dopamine, serotonin, and endorphins that will help make you feel better.

Do your best to find humor in your situation. Search for the ridiculous in everyday life, it's all around you. We find it useful to set time aside to watch shows, visit websites, or read comics, books, or articles that make you laugh. Up-and-coming comedians and long-term professional standups alike often post their performances on YouTube, which is a good place to find free comedy.

So, laugh at yourself. Laugh at the world. It may not truly be the best medicine, but it is a valuable tool in your healing arsenal. Lean into it.

Sunbeams grace the land
Nature awakens with joy
Sunlight's gift of life

A Sunny Disposition

Sunlight is known to boost your mood, mental health, vitamin D synthesis, energy levels, and sleep quality. According to a Harvard Medical School study, sunlight triggers the release of endorphins, reducing feelings of stress and anxiety while promoting relaxation.

You can acquire vitamin D through diet and supplementation, yet it's naturally boosted by sunlight. Symptoms of deficiency can include fatigue, depression, anxiety, irritability, hair loss, muscle weakness, cognitive decline, and a diminished immune system. Researchers estimate that as much as half the adult population in the United States may not be getting enough vitamin D. Chronic deficiency is linked to increased Alzheimer's risk and causes a decline in calcium and phosphorus absorption which in turn can lead to soft or brittle bones in adults and rickets in children.

So, a little sunlight can be a big thing when it comes to your mental and physical health, so long as you don't overdo it. Check with your care team, especially if you're undergoing radiation treatments, suffering from skin cancer, or taking medications that can cause sun sensitivity, but generally speaking 5 to 15 minutes can help you achieve the benefits of sun exposure at minimal risk. If you plan to spend any length of time outdoors you should apply a broad-spectrum sunscreen before you do.

We've found that spending a few minutes outside stretching on sunny mornings can do the trick. It gets you moving while simultaneously providing a little sun exposure. Further, closing your eyes, looking up, and feeling the sunlight on your face for a couple of minutes after stretching is cathartic. It's a great way to start your day.

Golden, crispy bite

Seasoned well and
deeply fried

Savory bliss found

Sour Your Sweet Tooth

While science has not verified a direct connection between sugar consumption and cancer, there is evidence of indirect linkage. For example, eating too much sugar can lead to weight gain, inflammation, and obesity, and there is a large body of evidence tying excess body fat to breast, colorectal, endometrial, esophageal, gall bladder, kidney, liver, mouth, pharynx, larynx, ovarian, pancreatic, prostate, and stomach cancers.

Cancer cells grow and multiply faster than healthy tissues, and that requires a lot of energy. Since this energy comes from sugar, or glucose in the bloodstream which is generated most easily from carbohydrates, there is a longstanding misconception that sugar causes cancer. It probably doesn't, at least not directly, but we all know that too much sugar isn't good for you. Since your body can convert fat and protein molecules into glucose too, there's really no downside to cutting back on sugar.

The average person in the United States consumes significantly more added sugar in their diet than doctors recommend for healthy people let alone for cancer patients. Although consensus is still emerging, and clinical trials have yet to definitively prove the connection, evidence from epidemiologic and preclinical studies demonstrates that excess sugar consumption can lead to development of cancer and to progression of the disease, even independent of the association between sugar and obesity.

Sugar can come from fruit (fructose), vegetables (glucose), dairy products (lactose), and refined sugar added to drinks or baked goods (sucrose). Excessive sugar intake can adversely affect your ability to utilize glucose efficiently, negatively impacting memory, cognitive abilities, and mood. It's addictive too.

We recommending reducing or eliminating sucrose, high-fructose corn syrup, and artificial sweeteners from your diet. Stop adding sugar to your coffee or tea. Cut out soda, candy bars, pastries, and overly refined foods. Even if this doesn't improve your condition or reduce your risk of reoccurrence, it will make you feel better for not eating it. So, sour your sweet tooth. You'll be healthier for doing it.

Whispers rise and curl

Steam dances from
hotter stones

Warmth in each
soft breath

Sauna

Lawrence has been lifting weights for... well pretty much as long as he can remember. After he hit the age of 45, he began having a harder and harder time recovering from heavy workouts without soreness, so he invested in a Finnish-style dry sauna. They're great for relieving muscle aches and pains when used properly. They also help with stiff joints, blood pressure, circulation, lung function, and immune health, and can even help stave off neurocognitive disease. You don't have to buy one, they're available at many health clubs and gyms.

Traditional saunas employ heat and steam to create an environment that raises your body temperature. Infrared saunas mimic this effect by using light to create heat. Either way, thermotherapy, otherwise known as passive heat therapy, can help restore and detoxify your body at the cellular level. That much is proven.

Researchers hypothesize that passive heat therapy such as using a sauna may help with cancer treatments too, such as by making radiation and chemotherapy more effective. They have found that infrared heat shrank tumors in mice, but that effect hasn't been replicated in humans yet insofar as we could find. There are clinical studies underway as of this writing, however, that are testing thermotherapy along with chemotherapy and other treatments designed to boost a patient's immune system to help fight cancer.

Using a sauna is not for everyone. For example, if you've been drinking, taking certain drugs, or using certain medications that inhibit your body's ability to control temperature you'll put yourself in danger. For most folks, however, they're relaxing and may even help with your condition. Check with your care team.

In shelter's embrace

*Calm and peace guard
weary hearts*

Safety's warm cocoon

Babies Love the Swaddle (and You do Too)

Babies love to be swaddled. Swaddling is the process of wrapping a newborn's body snugly in thin blanket or muslin wrap. It mimics the warmth and tightness of the womb, helping them feel secure. You see, infants are not accustomed to having their arms and legs sprawling outward. Simply put, swaddling is a known condition to the baby who finds themself in a new and unmanageable world.

You may want to mimic swaddling. For adults this is done with a weighted blanket. You can get many different versions of a weighted blanket. You can read product reviews online and find customers' stories of deep, restful sleep. This is due to a phenomenon called Deep Pressure Stimulation (DPS), which activates your body's relaxation response.

As martial artists we know as well as you do that when you control your mind, your body will follow. And, if you can control your body, your mind will follow. You don't need a multi-million-dollar study to know this, you've experienced it in your training. New mothers and midwives have been using the swaddling technique for centuries. You're not an infant, but your body is under attack by the cancer and treatment process. Soothe it and your mind will calm.

This is not a new insight, the mind-body connection. Swaddling works, even for adults. The first weighted blanket was invented in 1997 by Keith Zivalich when his daughter placed a beanie baby doll on his shoulder and he felt a calming sensation. The product was originally named the beanie blanket, but was later rebranded as the magic weighted blanket after customer feedback. The concept became popular nationwide in 2017 after a Kickstarter campaign for a competitor's product called the gravity blanket.

Weighted blankets are helpful for folks with anxiety, depression, autism, and other mental disorders, but not safe for very young children and individuals with sleep apnea because they can restrict airflow. Give one a try. You're likely to experience significantly better sleep quality, reduced anxiety, and less movement during sleep.

Silent tears fall down

Heartaches in the
quiet night

Pain whispers softly

Pain Changes Everything

Kris lay across his bed, breathing shallowly and quickly. It was two days past surgery. The doctor had made four, two-inch incisions down his side, between his ribs, to access his abdomen.

"You need pain meds."

Kris looked over at his son who was standing in the doorway with a concerned look on his face and replied, "No, just get me some Tylenol®."

There was no pause in his son's response, "Dad, you've just been stabbed four times. I'm getting the Oxy."

"Yeah, okay." Framed that way, it made sense to Kris.

Pain medication exists to be used. Don't be a tough guy, use them. It is unlikely you will become addicted. The doctors monitor these types of drugs tightly these days, especially opioids.

Depending on your treatments you might be prescribed anything from opioids to non-opioids, adjuvant analgesics, nerve blockers, or patient-controlled analgesia pumps. As your pain wanes you'll likely be prescribed lower doses or alternate medications. For now, when it really hurts, lean on the drugs that are designed to remove the pain and make your world better.

Here is one re-frame for you: Pain medications are tools, just like hammers or saws. You can't pound nails or cut wood without them. When you are done with your hammer or saw, you put it away. Do the same with your pain meds.

Chalk dust fills the air

Lessons dance on
eager minds

Wisdom passed like flame

Teaching and Training During Treatment

Martial arts training has been part of your life for years. You should be on the floor, teaching, or if you are a student training, you belong there. Don't let cancer stop you.

Now you may be thinking, "I don't know about that. I'm unable to do now what I once could." Or, you might be feeling, "I'm weak. I don't want to be seen like that." These are reasonable ideas, and we can certainly understand why you might think that way, but we disagree.

Let us present an alternative view. First, if your treatment is kicking your ass, as in on radiation therapy day, go ahead and stay home. That phase of treatment is tough. In other words, be reasonable. But, if you can get on the floor, do it. Your fellow martial artists are not going to perceive you as weak; they will recognize strength in your grit and determination and be inspired.

Martial arts practice benefits cancer patients both during and after treatment by improving musculoskeletal conditioning, flexibility, cognitive skills, lung capacity, and social function, among other things. It moderates anxiety and depression too. In fact, Kids Kicking Cancer and Cancer Warrior Martial Arts Program were both founded for that very reason. So, head to the training hall whenever you're able to do so.

Pace yourself. You may choose to show up for one class instead of for the full complement. You may need to take a break more often than normal. You may not be able to demonstrate at a high level, but you can point. Even if you're standing all by yourself on the edge of the mat, you still can watch, visualize, and continue to learn.

It feels good to put on your training uniform. It feels good to be amongst others who have a like mindset and goals. Also, being at the martial arts club brings some level of normalcy to an otherwise disrupted life. It may only be for an hour or two, but those moments are going to be wonderful.

We've done it, we recommend it, and we encourage you to get out there too. You will thank yourself for doing it.

Under bright lights' glare

Life and hope lie intertwined

Surgeon's steady heart

Quarantine

You have surgery scheduled. Know that your appointment is planned with care, coordinated just like a queue of commercial jets in landing formation at a busy airport like O'Hare in Chicago. O'Hare International is one of the busiest airports in the world, with an average of 2,520 planes taking off and landing every day. If you lose your position in the flight queue, you are going to have to circle back around and start over so that you won't interfere with the rest of the planes waiting to land.

Here is a fast way to get kicked out of the proverbial flight queue before surgery: Get sick. Catch a cold, get the flu, you're off the surgery list and sent to the back of the line. Your procedure is going to be rescheduled. Hospitals are busy, doctors have a lot going on, so getting sick for just a few days could mean weeks or months of delay in getting your operation. That means your healing process will be suspended. You'll miss out on vital surgery and the delay could be catastrophic for your recovery.

So, once you know you're in the proverbial flight queue waiting for surgery, protect your position with a self-imposed quarantine. Some hospitals ask you to isolate yourself and limit contact with others, but even if they don't it's a very good idea. Cancer patients are significantly more likely to get infections than regular folks because their immune systems are depressed from their condition or from the therapies used to treat it.

People will want to visit. Tell them, "Thank you, I'd love to see you, but I'm in pre-surgery quarantine." You'll want to go to dinner, do some shopping, or see a show, but surgery is far more important. Stay away from others, protect your health and stamina, and assure that your procedure will be done on time. A little inconvenience is a prudent precaution.

Calm beneath the storm

Inner refuge,
steady ground

Meditation's shield

Get a Hobby

There will be a lot of things that you can't control during your cancer recovery such as your diagnosis, progression of the disease, efficacy of your treatments, and severity of side effects, to name a few. Sure, you and your care team will make the best possible choices given your unique situation, but at times you'll feel like a leaf spinning through the rapids of a fast-flowing river. You know the direction you're headed, but have little ability to steer the course of exactly how you will get there.

A great way to bring more control into your life, one scientifically proven to have positive mental, physical, and social health benefits, is starting a new hobby (or leaning into one that you already enjoy and may not have done in a while). Building new skills, especially creative ones, can reduce stress, lighten your mood, moderate your blood pressure, and improve your focus and concentration.

Consider creative endeavors like photography, woodworking, painting, writing, knitting, pottery, music, knifemaking, embroidery, gardening, jewelry-making, or anything else where you are able to create something meaningful and lasting. The specific hobby you choose is less important than your level of engagement and sense of accomplishment from doing it.

Sure, your time and energy will likely be constrained during your treatment regimen, but it's important to invest in leisure activities to the extent feasible. A relaxing pastime can be a wonderful distraction from the rigors of treatment. Anything you can "get lost in" is fantastic. When shared with others, your hobby could lead to new friendships and camaraderie too.

So, get a hobby. The more meaningful it is to you, the better.

Elders' whispered tales

Ancient trees know
winds and time

Leaves fall, truths unveil

Follow Your Doctor's Advice

This chapter really shouldn't need to be written, you'd think it's kinda self-evident, but we're compelled to do so because upon driving into the parking garage at the Seattle Cancer Care Alliance facility in Burien, Washington, Lawrence saw someone smoking a cigarette through their stoma[5] while standing under a no-smoking sign. Twice. One was a crusty old World War II veteran in his late 90s or early 100s who apparently just didn't care any longer, but the other was a lady who appeared to be in her early- to mid-fifties. With an average life expectancy in the United States of about 80.2 years for females, that looked an awful lot like a slow-motion suicide attempt.

A study conducted by the Mayo Clinic estimated that only half of all cancer patients conscientiously follow instructions about taking their medications properly and on time. According to the National Institutes of Health, as many as 19% of cancer patients refuse chemotherapy, 15% decline hormone therapy, and 9.2% pass on first course treatments altogether. Of those who are treated, roughly 40% of patients increase their risks by misunderstanding, forgetting, ignoring, or neglecting their doctor's advice. And, few implement lifestyle changes necessary to keep their disease contained and reduce the chances that it will come back after treatments. That's mindboggling.

So, as we stated earlier on, be sure that you've found a great doctor, one who communicates clearly and effectively so that you can understand your unique situation, treatment options, and risks. Do your homework, ask good questions, actively listen, and then follow his or her advice. If you truly want to recover, there's no good excuse for not doing what your doctor tells you to do.

---

5   A stoma is an opening in the neck that allows a person to breathe properly after surgery to remove part or all of their larynx. This tracheostomy is often the result of laryngeal, mouth, or oropharyngeal cancer caused by smoking cigarettes.

Gardener's kind hands

Nurture blooms
with patient care

Flowers grow in trust

Paying for Care

Cancer is expensive. According to the American Cancer Society there are roughly 1.9 million new cases diagnosed each year in the United States alone, and patients spend an estimated $5.6 billion annually on out-of-pocket expenses associated with their diagnosis, treatment, and recovery. Depending on how much if any insurance you bought, what type of insurance you have, how early your illness was discovered, whether treatments are in- or out of network, co-payment requirements, outlay caps, and the like, you can expect to spend upwards of $150,000 for care.

That's a lot of money, but thankfully, you don't have to go it alone. Speak with your care team, they can help connect you with patient advocacy organizations, treatment centers, cancer non-profits, drug companies, and religious institutions who may be able to provide financial assistance. There are state and federal government programs that help with medical bills, transportation costs, and living expenses. They can even replace some or all of your lost wages if you are unable to work during treatments too.

Beyond your care team, there are numerous online sources of data that can help you connect with resources and assistance. A useful one is CancerCare's "helping hand," a database you can search to discover practical help and financial aid from organizations in your local area. Here's the link: https://www.cancercare.org/helpinghand.

If you're willing to make your condition public, consider starting a GoFundMe or GiveSendGo site to raise money to help defray your treatment costs. You'll be pleasantly surprised by how generous folks can be. CaringBridge (https://www.caringbridge.org/) is a non-profit platform that helps you coordinate communication with people who you wish to know about your condition and progress. They can provide support in asking for help too.

Yes, cancer is expensive. Understand your benefits, arrange payment plans if you must, and never be afraid to ask for help. There are ton of resources out there for you.

Brush strokes on canvas
Colors blend stories unfold
Art breathes life anew

Tattoo You?

Cancer survivors often use tattoos to camouflage surgical or radiation scars and commemorate their healing journey. If you still have a compromised immune system after your treatments or are undergoing chemotherapy, you're better off taking a pass on having a tattoo done. You're not ready yet. Typically, you'll want it until after you're fully healed so that the tattoo won't interfere with your treatments or create any elevated risks to your health. If you're considering getting one, check with your care team first.

Some tattoo artists specialize in working with cancer patients, and your doctor might be able to point you to one. A few considerations: It goes without saying, but tattoos are permanent, so put a lot of thought into it and choose your design wisely. Laser tattoo removal is no fun. Even more importantly, choose your artist and studio with care. You risk infection, allergic reaction, or contracting a nasty blood-borne pathogen like hepatitis or tetanus if you pick a place that isn't sufficiently sanitary and well-run.

Not all tattoo artists are comfortable or experienced with tattooing over scar tissue, if that's what you'd like done. You may be able to find someone who specializes in working with cancer survivors through the Alliance of Professional Tattooists, an association that promotes health, safety, and professionalism in the industry. Another option is the Tattoo Artists Guild.

Even though they're injected into your skin, tattoo inks aren't regulated by the FDA. Some contain azo dyes, which aren't harmful when they're chemically intact but may become carcinogenic if they're exposed to bacteria or ultraviolet light and break down. Use caution and ask questions before having anything done.

Know that tattoos must be kept clean and dry while they're healing. Usually, the artist will recommend washing with antibacterial soap and applying a thin layer of antibiotic ointment or coconut oil on a daily basis until it has fully healed. Never use a hot tub with a fresh tattoo, that invites infection.

Waves crash on the shore

Endless rhythm,
timeless beat

Nature's repeat dance

It May Not Be Over When It's Over

Even after you've finished your treatment regimen, your ordeal may not be over yet. Depending on what you were diagnosed with and what kinds of treatments were used, many cancers have a nasty habit of coming back to haunt you again within the first two to five years after treatment. Ovarian cancer and glioblastoma (a rare brain cancer), for example, have a very high reoccurrence rate, whereas noninvasive breast cancer and Hodgkin lymphoma rarely return. The statistics really don't matter, because this is a giant case of "it depends," but it's best to be prepared just in case.

Certain treatment regimens can cause secondary cancers too. For example, acute myelogenous leukemia, acute lymphocytic leukemia, myelodysplastic syndromes, thyroid cancer, and wide variety of solid tumors can stem from chemotherapy and radiation treatments. The risks of this happening increase with higher drug doses, longer treatment times, and higher dose-intensities. If you had an allogeneic transplant, you risk graft-versus-host disease, which isn't another cancer but requires immunosuppressants, steroids, and targeted drug therapies to remediate. Your care team will monitor for these sorts of complications, of course, and you'll undoubtedly get a variety of scans and blood tests to minimize the risk and keep everything on track.

Hopefully your recovery will be complete after your first set of treatments, but you can't count on it. You can, however, increase your odds of not needing to re-undergo treatment by scheduling regular follow-up screenings and ongoing visits with your care team, working with a naturopathic oncologist, and making healthy lifestyle changes. Since only about five to ten percent of cancers are caused by inherited gene mutations, if you exercise regularly, eat "real" food, maintain a healthy bodyweight, limit alcohol, protect yourself from the sun, and stay away from tobacco you'll be making a tremendous difference. That's your best way of safeguarding your health long term.

If your cancer does return, think of it like a belt test you failed. It's nothing more than a bump in the road. Dust yourself off, pick yourself up, prepare as best you can, and try it again. Sure, a do-over is no fun, but it's not the end of your journey. You're a martial artist, you've got this.

Forked path in forest

Decisions mark
the journey

Choices shape our fate

Conclusion

"Rode hard and put away wet," is a phrase that Kris would sometimes hear from his father. It originated way back when folks relied on horses for their daily transportation and used one to the point of exhaustion.

Kris's father used that phrase to describe how he felt after working a long day for another person. That idiom is based on riding a horse hard, overworking it, and then leaving it in a bad state by not wiping it down and grooming it properly afterward. It implies exhaustion, a worn-out look, and habitual misuse.

At your cancer care facility, you are going to see a lot of people who have been rode hard and put away wet. Obesity is common. Mobility aids like walkers, canes, and wheelchairs, and breathing aids like portable oxygen concentrators are often observed. You can tell that many of these folks came from a long history of poor choices, decisions made daily that incrementally added up to them finding themselves in need of cancer care.

Sure, genetic factors and environmental pollutants play an important role, but things you can control like smoking, physical inactivity, unhealthy diet, excessive alcohol consumption, and chronic inflammation are common precursors of cancer. Most of the folks in the waiting room at your cancer care facility let themselves go long before finding themselves in need of medical attention.

Others don't fit this description. They looked and felt healthy, hence were shocked when their cancer showed up. They are the exception. You are too, you're the exception. Never forget that.

You are different. You have martial arts discipline. Muscle tone, mobility, lung capacity, and flexibility are but a few of the benefits that you have gained over your time in the training hall. You have grit, determination, and mental discipline. You are not like most of the people you'll see in the reception room at the cancer care center. Not at all. It is important that you know this and lean into it.

With your distinctiveness comes opportunity, and a higher level of responsibility. You can lift others up, the folks who see themselves as victims, the ones who can't differentiate between their self-identify and the disease they've contracted. You know you're not a victim, you know you're ready for your fight, but most of the folks around you cannot see this in themselves. They wallow in misery.

Get to know the folks in the waiting room a little. Oftentimes you'll be on the same treatment schedule, so you'll see them repeatedly. Listen to their stories, understand what they're going through. Active listening has value, even if you don't say much. Humans are social animals; we need to be heard. So, have a chat of encouragement with the other patients around you while waiting for your appointment whenever you can.

"Nice to see you again. You look good today. How are you feeling?"

Share fist-bump in passing, "Stay strong."

"Is this your wife? You are lucky to have such support."

You get the idea… Keep it upbeat. Don't be weird or disingenuous when talking to others, but do talk to them.

Because of your training, your skills, and your discipline, you're in a different place than most of those around you. Whenever you can, give a tip of the cap in the direction of others who are less fortunate. Through their choices, or the cards they were dealt, they were ridden hard and put away wet. You weren't, even if some days you might feel like it.

Stay strong, and be well,

Kris   Lawrence

"Today we fight. Tomorrow, we fight. The day after, we fight. And if this disease plans on whipping us, it better bring a lunch, 'cause it's gonna have a long day doing it."

———————————————

Jim Beaver

Bibliography

Books:

- Antonicelli, Frank III. *Know Your Enemy: A Guidebook for Your Cancer Journey*. NY: Page Publishing, 2016.
- Buckman, Robert, MD. *Cancer is a Word, Not a Sentence: A Practical Guide to Help You Through the First Few Weeks*. NY: Firefly Books, Ltd., 2006
- Emerson, Nancy, Susan Moonan, and Terri Schinazi. *Finding the Can in Cancer*. NC: Lulu Press, 2007
- Halverson-Boyd, Glenna, and Lisa K. Hunter. *Dancing in Limbo: Making Sense of Life After Cancer*. CA: Jossey-Bass Publishers, 1995.
- Holtz, Michael. *It's Not Harder Than Cancer: The Mindsets You Need to Survive and Thrive After Serious Illness*. SC: CreateSpace Independent Publishing, 2015.
- Kalanithi, Paul. *When Breath Becomes Air*. NY: Random House, 2016.
- Levine, Stephen. *A Year to Live: How to Live This Year as If It Were Your Last*. NY: Harmony Books, 1997.
- Potts, Bill C. *Up for the Fight: How to Advocate for Yourself as You Battle Cancer from a Five-Time Survivor*. Vancouver BC: Page Two Publishing, 2022.
- Rubiana, Margaret. *I'm Dead, Now What? Planner—Important Information about My Belongings, Business Affairs, and Wishes*. NY: Peter Pauper Press, 2015.
- Wolters, Lynda. *Voices of Cancer: What We Really Want, What We Really Need—Insights for Patients and the People Supporting Them*. VA: Mascot Books, 2019.
- Zavaleta, Beverly A, M.D. *Braving Chemo: What to Expect, How to Prepare, and How to Get Through It*. OR: Sugar Plum Press, LLC. 2019.

Articles:

- Abernethy, E. R., Campbell, G. P., and Pentz, R. D. Why Many Oncologists Fail to Share Accurate Prognoses: They Care Deeply for Their Patients. *Cancer.* March 15, 2020.

- Andrade C., Radhakrishnan R. Prayer and Healing: A Medical and Scientific Perspective on Randomized Controlled Trials. *Indian Journal of Psychiatry.* October – December, 2009.

- Bohlmeijer, E. T., Kraiss, J. T., Watkins, P., et al. Promoting Gratitude as a Resource for Sustainable Mental Health: Results of a 3-Armed Randomized Controlled Trial up to 6 Months Follow-up. *Journal of Happiness Studies.* May 7, 2020.

- Boyes, Alice Ph.D. What Is Psychological Shock? And 5 Tips for Coping. *Psychology Today,* March 6, 2018

- Brown, M. T., Bussell, J. K. Medication adherence: WHO cares? *Mayo Clinic Proceedings.* April, 2011 Apr.

- Cross, M. P., Acevedo, A. M., Leger, K. A., and Pressman, S. D. How and Why Could Smiling Influence Physical Health? *Health Psychology Review.* June 17, 2023.

- Cui, J., Ding, R., Liu, H., et al. Trends in the incidence and survival of cancer in individuals aged 55 years and older in the United States, 1975–2019. *BMC Public Health.* January 3, 2024

- De Cabo, Rafael, Ph.D. and Mark P. Mattson, Ph.D. Effects of Intermittent Fasting on Health, Aging, and Disease. *The New England Journal of Medicine.* December 25, 2019.

- Epner M., Yang P., Wagner R.W., and Cohen L. Understanding the Link between Sugar and Cancer: An Examination of the Preclinical and Clinical Evidence. *Cancers.* December 8, 2022.

- Gao W., Xie W., Xie W., Jiang C., Kang Z., and Liu N. An Enriched Environment Promotes Cognitive Recovery and Cerebral Blood Flow in Aged Mice Under Sevoflurane Anesthesia. *National Genomics Data Center Folia Neuropathol.* August 21, 2024.

- Gillette, Hope, Ari Howard, and Sheel Patel, M.D. Your Guide to Assembling a Personalized Cancer Team. *Healthline.* July 11, 2024.

- Hughes, C. E. Prayer and Healing. A Case Study. *Journal of Holistic Nursing.* September 15, 1997.
- Hussain J., Cohen M. Clinical Effects of Regular Dry Sauna Bathing: A Systematic Review. *Evidence Based Complementary Alternative Medicine.* April 24, 2018.
- Jaffe, Eric. The Psychological Study of Smiling. *Association for Psychological Science.* February 11, 2011.
- Johnstone, C., and Rich, S. E. Bleeding in Cancer Patients and Its Treatment: A Review. *Annals of Palliative Medicine.* April 7, 2018.
- Kando-Pineda, C. How the Federal Trade Commission is Fighting Cancer Treatment Scams. *Journal of Oncology Practice.* January, 2010.
- Keegan, Theresa, Ph.D., M.S., Renata Abrahao, Ph.D., M.D., M.S., and Elysia M. Alvarez, M.D., M.P.H. Survival Trends Among Adolescents and Young Adults Diagnosed with Cancer in the United States: Comparisons with Children and Older Adults. *Journal of Clinical Oncology.* October 26, 2023.
- Laukkanen, J. A. and Kunutsor, S. K. The Multifaceted Benefits of Passive Heat Therapies for Extending the Health Span: A Comprehensive Review with a Focus on Finnish Sauna. *Temperature° Medical Physiology.* February 25, 2024.
- Lee, S.H., Zhao, L., Park, S., Moore, L.V., et. al. High Added Sugars Intake Among US Adults: Characteristics, Eating Occasions, and Top Sources. *Nutrients.* June 4, 2023.
- Ligibel, Jennifer A., M.D., Kari Bohlke, Sc.D., Ann M. May, Ph. D., Steven K. Clinton, M.D., Ph.D., et. al. Exercise, Diet, and Weight Management During Cancer Treatment: ASCO Guideline. *Journal of Clinical Oncology.* May 16, 2022.
- Lindsay, E. K., Young, S., and Creswell, J. D. Mindfulness Training Fosters a Positive Outlook During Acute Stress: A Randomized Controlled Trial. *Emotion.* November, 2024.
- Louie D., Brook K., Frates E. The Laughter Prescription: A Tool for Lifestyle Medicine. *American Journal of Lifestyle Medicine.* June 23, 2016.
- Mead, M.N. Benefits of Sunlight: A Bright Spot for Human Health. *Environmental Health Perspectives.* April – May, 2008.

- Milazzo, S., Horneber, M. Laetrile Treatment for Cancer. *The Cochrane Database of Systematic Reviews.* April 28, 2015.
- Mortada E. M. Evidence-Based Complementary and Alternative Medicine in Current Medical Practice. *The Cureus Journal of Medial Science.* January, 2024
- Nair S., Sagar M., Sollers J., 3rd, Consedine N., Broadbent E. Do Slumped and Upright Postures Affect Stress Responses? A Randomized Trial. *American Psychological Association Health Psychology.* June, 2015.
- O'Brien, Scott. Faith and Healing. *Harvard Medical School,* December 3, 2013.
- Owens, Lisa Viani. Good Posture is Important for Physical and Mental Health. *San Francisco State University News.* December 15, 2017.
- Palosky, Craig and Larry Levitt. Kaiser/Harvard Survey Highlights Problems in the Health Care System Through the Experiences of People with Cancer. *USA Today.* November 1, 2006.
- Pressman, S. D., Matthews, K. A., Cohen, S., et. al. Association of Enjoyable Leisure Activities with Psychological and Physical Well-Being. *Psychosomatic Medicine.* September, 2009.
- Raman, Ryan, M.S., and Angelica Balingit, M.D. How to Safely Get Vitamin D From Sunlight. *Healthline.* November 26, 2024.
- Rosenbaum, Ernest H., M.D. and Isadora R. Rosenbaum, M.A. The Will to Live. *Stanford Center for Integrative Medicine.* July 1, 2019.
- Sur, D., Sabarimurugan, S., and Advani, S. The Effects of Martial Arts on Cancer-Related Fatigue and Quality of Life in Cancer Patients. *International Journal of Environmental Research and Public Health.* June 6, 2021.
- Tanaka, Y., Matsuo K., Yuzuriha S., Yan H., and Nakayama J. Non-Thermal Cytocidal Effect of Infrared Irradiation on Cultured Cancer Cells Using Specialized Device. *Cancer Science.* June, 2010.
- Toolis, Brittany. Seattle Cancer Patients Face Blackmail Threats After Recent Fred Hutch Data Breach. *KIRO 7 News.* December 7, 2023.

- Vaish A, Grossmann T, Woodward A. Not all emotions are created equal: the negativity bias in social-emotional development. *Psychological Bulletin.* May, 2008.
- Ying, Chen, Olivia I. Okereke, Eric S. Kim, et. Al. Gratitude and Mortality Among Older US Female Nurses. *Journal of the American Medical Association Psychiatry.* July 3, 2024
- Yu, B. B., Huang L., Tiwari R. C., Feuer E. J., and Johnson K. A. Modelling population-based cancer survival trends by using join point models for grouped survival data. *Journal of the Royal Statistical Society.* April, 2009

Websites:

- American Cancer Society (https://www.cancer.org/)
- Aplastic Anemia & MDS International Foundation (https://www.aamds.org/)
- CaringBridge (https://www.caringbridge.org/)
- CancerCare's Helping Hand database (https://www.cancercare.org/helpinghand)
- Cancer Hope Network (https://cancerhopenetwork.org/)
- Cancer Lifeline (https://cancerlifeline.org/)
- Cancer Pathways (https://cancerpathways.org/)
- Cancer Research UK (https://www.cancerresearchuk.org/)
- CDC's National Center for Health Statistics (https://www.cdc.gov/nchs/index.html)
- City of Hope Blog: What you Should Know About Tattoos and Cancer (https://www.cancercenter.com/community/blog/2023/02/what-you-should-know-about-tattoos-and-cancer)
- EmergingMed Clinical Trial Navigation Service (https://app.emergingmed.com/emed/home)
- Fred Hutchinson Cancer Research Center (https://www.fredhutch.org/en.html)
- MediFind (https://www.medifind.com/)
- National Breast Cancer Foundation (https://www.nationalbreastcancer.org/)

- NCI Talking about Complementary and Alternative Medicine with Health Care Providers Workbook (https://cam.cancer.gov/health_information/talking_about_cam.htm)
- Oncology Association of Naturopathic Physicians (https://www.oncanp.org/)
- Prostate Cancer Foundation (https://www.pcf.org/)
- Psychology Today (https://www.psychologytoday.com/us)
- Statista (https://www.statista.com/)
- The American Society of Clinical Oncology (https://www.asco.org/)
- The Center for Information and Study on Clinical Research Participation (https://www.ciscrp.org/)
- The Lancet (https://www.thelancet.com/journals/lancet/home)
- The Leukemia & Lymphoma Society (https://www.lls.org/)
- The Mayo Clinic (https://www.mayoclinic.org/)
- The Myelodysplastic Syndromes Foundation (https://www.mds-foundation.org/)
- The National Cancer Institute (https://www.cancer.gov/)
- The National Institutes of Health (https://www.nih.gov/)

Videos:

- Anatomy of a Cancer Scam (https://www.cancer.gov/about-cancer/managing-care/using-trusted-resources/health-info-online)
- Clinical Trial Phases (https://www.youtube.com/watch?v=q9Zc27cL-FY)
- Complementary and Alternative Medicine for Cancer (https://www.youtube.com/watch?v=zPgUiBPp9mY)
- Considering a Cancer Clinical Trial (https://youtu.be/kh1IVFbo-VQ)
- Understanding Charitable Patient Assistance Programs (https://www.youtube.com/watch?v=60YnL7FRUHI)
- Why Cancer Clinical Trials Are So Important (https://www.youtube.com/watch?v=5-Sx8VqhPhs)
- Your Rights and Protections in a Clinical Trial (https://www.youtube.com/watch?v=OmQjTbBeu7w)

About the Authors

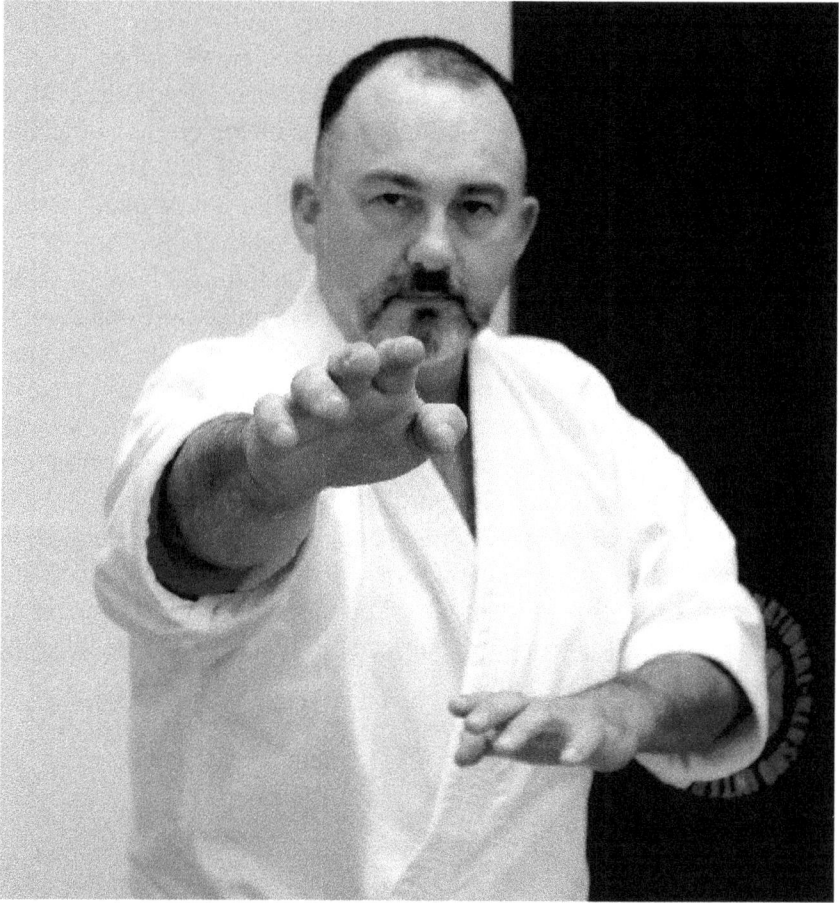

Kris Wilder

Kris was inducted into the U.S. Martial Arts Hall of Fame in 2018. He runs the *Cheney Karate Academy*, a frequent destination for practitioners from around the world which also serves the local community. He has earned black belt rankings in three styles, karate, judo, and taekwondo, and often travels to conduct seminars across the United States, Canada, and Europe. His book, *The Way of Sanchin*

Kata, was translated into Japanese, a rare honor for a Western karate practitioner.

A Nationally Board-Certified Life Coach and prolific author, Kris has lectured at Washington State University and Susquehanna University and served as an advisor for the Eastern Washington University Karate Club.

He spent about 15 years in the political and public affairs arena, working for campaigns from the local to national level. During this consulting career, he was periodically on staff for elected officials. His work also involved lobbying and corporate affairs. And, he was also a member of The Order of St. Francis (OSF), one of many active Apostolic Christian Orders.

Kris is the bestselling author of 34 books, including a Beverly Hills Book Award and Presidential Prize winner, a Living Now Book Award winner, a USA Best Book Awards winner, a National Indie Excellence Awards winner, three Independent Press Award winners, a Next Generation Indie Book Awards winner, and two Eric Hoffer award nominees. He has been interviewed on CNN, FOX, The Huffington Post, Thrillist, Nickelodeon, Howard Stern, and more.

Kris lives in Cheney, Washington. He was diagnosed with metastasized stage 4 adenocarcinoma, a type of cancer that starts in the glands that line your organs. You can contact him directly at kriswilder@kriswilder.com or connect on social media at: https://linktr.ee/KrisWilder.

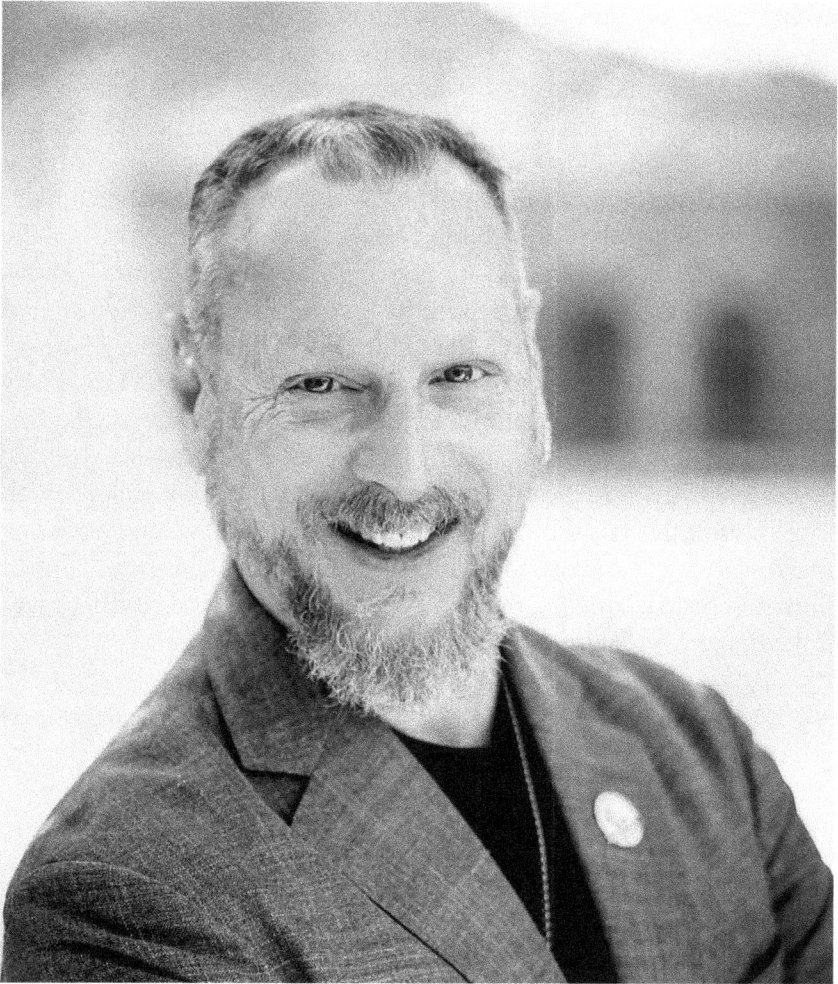

Lawrence A. Kane

Lawrence is Head of Procurement at a leading diversified financial services company in the United States. He was inducted into the SIG Sourcing Supernova Hall of Fame in 2018 for visionary leadership in strategic sourcing, procurement, supplier innovation, and digital transformation. In 2023 he earned an EPIC Award for lifetime achievements in indirect procurement from ProcureCon.

Over the course of his career, he institutionalized world-class practices that earned the prestigious Global Excellence in Outsourcing award from IAOP and six Future of Sourcing innovation awards from SIG, among other honors. He regularly advances thought leadership as a keynote speaker at industry conferences.

Lawrence has been studying and teaching martial arts since 1970, including a wide variety of traditional Asian styles, medieval swordsmanship, modern combatives, and close-quarters combat. The bestselling author of 31 books, he has been a guest on nationally syndicated and local radio shows (e.g., The Jim Bohannon Show, Biz Talk Radio), television programs (e.g., Fox Morning News), and podcasts (e.g., Art of Procurement, Negotiations Ninja Podcast, Sourcing Industry Landscape), and has also been interviewed by reporters from *Information Week, Le Matin, CPO Strategy, Forbes, Jissen,* and *Computerworld,* among other publications.

Lawrence lives in Seattle, Washington. He was diagnosed with myelodysplasia syndrome, a rare cancer that occurs when your bone marrow doesn't produce enough healthy blood cells. You can contact him directly at lakane@ix.netcom.com or connect on LinkedIn (www. linkedin.com/in/lawrenceakane).

Explore More Books from The Authors

Kris Wilder and Lawrence Kane are the bestselling, award-winning authors of *Musashi's Dokkodo, The Little Black Book of Violence, 10 Rules of Karate, Dude, The World's Gonna Punch You in the Face,* and *Martial Arts and Your Life,* among numerous other titles. Discover more below…

Kris Wilder

Lawrence A. Kane

www.ingramcontent.com/pod-product-compliance
Lightning Source LLC
Chambersburg PA
CBHW060501280326
41933CB00014B/2822